The Hashimoto's 4-Week Plan

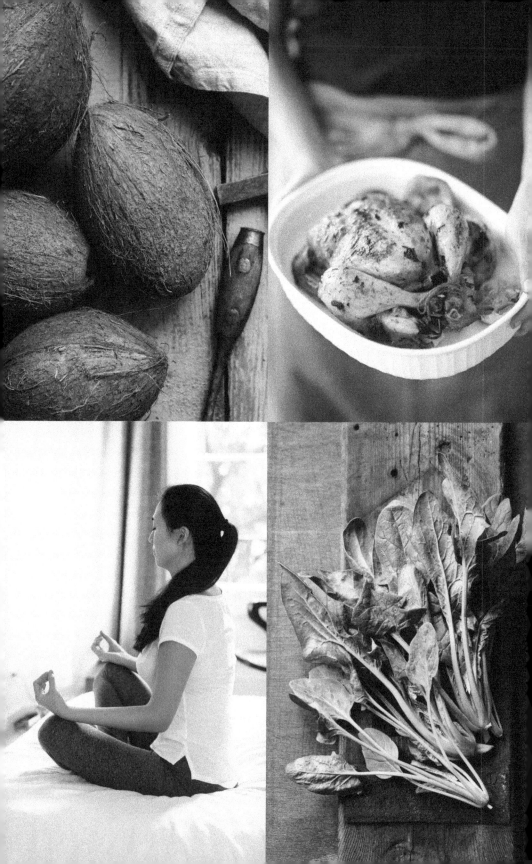

The

HASHIMOTO'S
4-WEEK PLAN

*A Holistic Guide to
Treating Hypothyroidism*

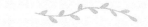

KAREN FRAZIER

Foreword by
Sara Peternell, MNT

SONOMA
PRESS

For Etta, my kitchen mentor,
and Jim, who has always encouraged
me to listen to my inner voice.

My Invitation to You

Hashimoto's disease is complex. It disrupts your bodily functions and toys with your emotions. Outsiders may not recognize your challenges because you don't "look sick." Struggling to understand your symptoms can cause you to doubt the validity of your disease—and yourself.

If you're like me, then you've probably received much unsolicited advice regarding your sudden weight fluctuations, plunging energy levels, and bouts of depression and anxiety.

- "Eat less, move more."
- "Just buck up and do it."
- "Focus on the positive."

Such well-meaning advice can be unhelpful and discouraging. You've probably tried to follow it; I know I did, and ended up feeling like a failure for not living up to other people's expectations. I thought of succumbing to my disease, but my inner voice kicked in and gave me some better ideas.

You, too, have a powerful inner voice, and I encourage you to listen to it. You, alone, know your strengths and limitations and, most importantly, your own body.

Throughout this book you will find inspiration and ideas to help you tune in to your inner wisdom. You'll learn to manage your Hashimoto's holistically, on *your* terms. This book is an invitation to return to yourself and discover the inner power that can lead you to wellness.

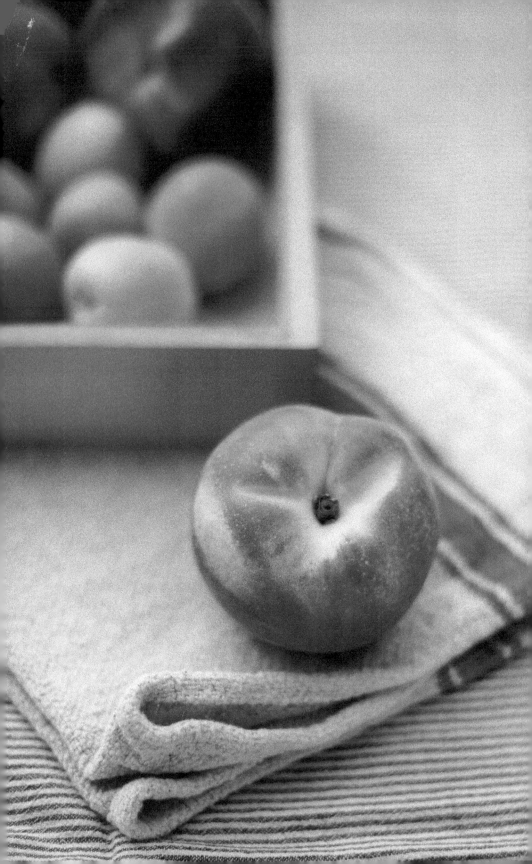

CONTENTS

FOREWORD

The beginning of my journey with Hashimoto's will probably sound familiar to you. In my 20s, I suddenly felt like an old woman. I had aches and pains. I was tired. And after rapidly gaining weight despite being petite my entire life, I was mildly depressed.

Like many Americans, I grew up on a less than healthy diet. I didn't know there was another way to eat. From the time I was a little girl, I had been plagued with digestive complaints, but no one ever wondered what could be wrong with me. Doctors just told me I had irritable bowel syndrome, and family members said I was "emotional."

Amazingly, despite having no clear intention to do so, I began a healing journey when I devoted myself to yoga as both a student and instructor. Further study about the human body led me to a career in holistic nutrition. While studying to become a Master Nutrition Therapist, I finally uncovered what was wrong with me. At the age of 24, I asked my doctor for a full panel of thyroid tests. Although my doctor said I only needed a low dose of antidepressant medication, she acquiesced, and with my antithyroid antibody levels in the thousands—yes, thousands—I was diagnosed with Hashimoto's thyroiditis.

My prescribed treatment plan was simple: take medication for the rest of my life to "control symptoms." Like so many sufferers of Hashimoto's, I struggled to feel better with this conventional approach. When I was 30, I was diagnosed with celiac disease. After suffering three miscarriages before having my two beautiful children, I became convinced that my seemingly unrelated health issues were connected to my thyroid—and its dysfunction.

To better manage my disease, I took it upon myself to study the thyroid, the endocrine system, and the extensive nutritional needs of the body. My final project for nutrition school was an in-depth protocol of an anti-inflammatory food plan to reverse autoimmune disease. I devoted my nutrition practice, Family Nutrition Services, to helping people like me learn more about their natural options for managing Hashimoto's through food and supplements. If you have the means to do so, I encourage you to find a qualified nutrition practitioner who can help you develop your own individualized nutrition plan. (This is especially true if you wish to take supplements, since their misuse can inadvertently worsen symptoms in some people.)

I am so happy to say that today, in my 40s, I am healthier than I have ever been. My antibodies are back within normal levels, and multiple doctors have told me my Hashimoto's is now in remission. They have even asked me what I am doing to make that possible. Clearly, the medical community has a long way to go in understanding this complex disease. Fortunately, there is much that we do know, and I am living proof that following the wonderful self-care practices and healthy eating guidelines like the ones outlined in this book can go a long way in managing symptoms.

It took me years of trial and error and in-depth nutrition studies to find my way to better health. I wish I had had *The Hashimoto's 4-Week Plan* fifteen years ago when I was first diagnosed. I look forward to recommending it to my own clients who come to me seeking nutritional advice for managing their Hashimoto's, and I hope this book helps you find much needed relief from your symptoms, too.

Sara Peternell, MNT

INTRODUCTION

I f you picked up this book, you're probably seeking better health along your Hashimoto's journey. You may have lingering symptoms despite your medications or other medical interventions. It can be frustrating to follow your doctor's instructions and still not feel well. However, in the case of most chronic illnesses like Hashimoto's, there isn't a one-size-fits-all solution. That's why this book contains a host of suggested lifestyle and diet interventions to help you develop a personalized plan allowing you to achieve optimal health. The book's title suggests it is a four-week plan, but you are free to stretch it for as long as you wish, or for as long as it takes to be effective. Over the long term, the goal is to establish new lifestyle habits that will help you live the best life you can with Hashimoto's.

How do I know all of this? I, too, have Hashimoto's disease. Although I didn't have official diagnoses until well into my forties, I'd known for more than 20 years that something was amiss. The multitude of symptoms I experienced—weight gain, fatigue, gastrointestinal distress, migraines, and muscle pain—were impossible to ignore, forcing me to make tough choices.

Where I had once been an active person, I no longer had the physical stamina to live an active life. I changed jobs from a physically arduous position as a personal trainer and fitness instructor to a more sedentary occupation. And while the physical and emotional aspects of Hashimoto's took a toll on many areas of my life, my lifestyle change gave me the time to develop many of my current passions, including writing, which is my beloved career today.

I also learned other valuable lessons: to put myself first, to develop a sense of self apart from my physical appearance and limitations, to trust my intuitive wisdom about my body and my health, and to educate myself and fiercely advocate for myself as a healthcare consumer. These have all been important factors in arriving at where I am today: feeling healthier than I have in years.

Well before my diagnoses, I intuitively understood dietary modifications might help me feel better, and I made various changes to see what helped. I followed many different diets with mixed results. However, it wasn't until I started eating a clean anti-inflammatory diet, free of processed foods, dairy, and gluten, that I started to notice a change. While many of my symptoms improved, others persisted. I realized lifestyle modifications were in order, as well. I needed to be kinder to myself physically, spiritually, and emotionally, so I changed how I slept, managed stress, exercised, and talked to myself. I learned to find a balance between my needs and the needs of others.

I share my nutrition knowledge and lifestyle modifications within this book along with 78 tasty recipes, many of which can be made in less than 15 minutes. These recipes will make it easier to integrate healthful foods into your Hashimoto's four-week plan.

Making the lifestyle modifications and eating the foods recommended in this book, in combination with the right medications and support team, have made a world of difference in how I feel and act. I have more energy than I've had in years, and I've lost more than 125 pounds. I sleep well, and am often pain-free. While different people may experience different results, I hope this book will inspire you to think of new ways to be kinder to yourself, listen to your wise inner voice, and improve the quality of your physical and emotional life.

I am honored to be part of your journey.

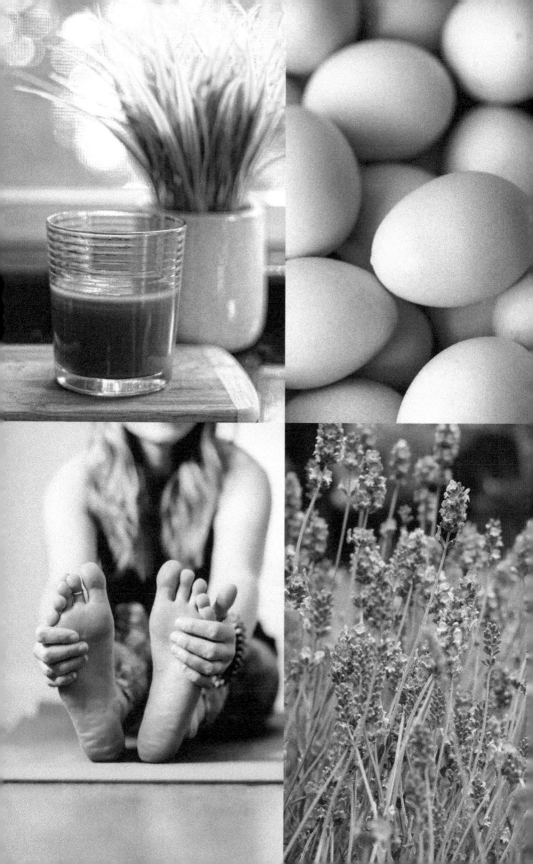

PART 1

The Road to Better Health and Well-Being

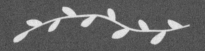

1

BIG PICTURE BASICS

Welcome to the world of Hashimoto's thyroiditis, a chronic condition that affects virtually every cell in your body. Discovered by a Japanese medical scientist named Hakaru Hashimoto in 1912, Hashimoto's thyroiditis was among the first to be categorized as an autoimmune disease in the early twentieth century. Today, it's believed to affect as many as 5 percent of adults in the Western world and about 15 million Americans, according to *Medical News Today*.

A diagnosis of Hashimoto's disease brings as much confusion and questions as it does relief. If you're like me and many other sufferers, long-standing symptoms have led you on a wild-goose chase for years. Fortunately, with diagnosis comes hope, and a chance to learn new ways to take care of your health and regain the sense of normalcy you may have feared lost. In the pages that follow, I'll help you get on the path to better health with Hashimoto's.

UNDERSTANDING THE IMMUNE SYSTEM

Your immune system exists to help your body stay healthy. It is a wonderfully intricate system designed to fight foreign invaders and keep all your bodily systems humming along in good health. When it works, it is a beautiful thing. However, when something goes awry, your immune system can turn on your body, a condition known as autoimmunity, and cause a chronic form of illness known as autoimmune disease.

According to the *Merck Manual*, "The immune system sometimes malfunctions, interpreting the body's own tissues as foreign and producing antibodies (called autoantibodies) or immune cells that target and attack particular cells or tissues of the body. This response is called an autoimmune reaction. It results in inflammation and tissue damage."

Making sense of this intricate dance between immune responses, cells and antigens, and inflammation provides a fuller understanding of how the entire immune system is meant to work and, therefore, how it is impeded by autoimmune disease.

Immune Response

When your body is faced with foreign invaders, such as germs or other disease-causing organisms (pathogens), your immune system kicks in. Ideally, your immune system will fight off pending infection, and you won't get sick. However, in some cases, your initial immune response isn't strong enough, and you get sick anyway. In those cases, your immune system offers additional responses to clear the pathogens from your body as quickly as possible. Examples of these immune responses include:

- Fever to burn out disease-causing organisms
- Vomiting or diarrhea to expel germs from the body quickly
- Inflammation to localize and eliminate invading pathogens to promote healing

White Blood Cells

Your white blood cells, also called leukocytes, serve as one of the immune system's primary modes of defense against infectious organisms. There are two major subtypes of white blood cells circulating throughout the body. One (phagocytes) is released to fight off infectious agents. The other (lymphocytes) recognizes previous foreign substances, seeking to destroy them when they reappear.

White blood cells serve as a sort of police force in your body. They circulate through blood and lymphatic vessels, monitoring what's going on. When they detect the presence of a disease-causing invader, the cells respond by destroying the infectious agents. In many cases, such as chicken pox, the body creates antigens, which are fragments of proteins the white blood cells can recognize and for which they can create antibodies. These antibodies will always recognize and destroy any pathogens from that disease when they appear again, conferring a lifetime of immunity to that disease.

Autoimmune Disease

While the ever-vigilant immune system is on constant alert for disease-causing organisms, occasionally something goes haywire. In the case of autoimmune disease, the immune system begins to respond to normal tissue as if it were a harmful foreign invader, thereby launching a defensive attack against normal, healthy tissue. This results in the destruction of healthy tissue. In the case of Hashimoto's thyroiditis, your friendly thyroid has come under siege by a mistaken and misdirected immune response. With each firebomb received, the thyroid functions less and less efficiently, causing a plethora of symptoms mentioned earlier.

According to the U.S. National Library of Medicine, several results may occur as the immune system continues to attack the body, including:

- Destruction of healthy body tissue (in Hashimoto's, the thyroid)
- Changes in the function of the affected organ (in Hashimoto's, changing how your body manufactures and releases thyroid hormones)

- Abnormalities in the organ's size (in Hashimoto's, an enlarged thyroid, called a goiter, is a common symptom)

Hashimoto's is just one of more than 80 types of autoimmune diseases that occur in the human population, but it is among the most prevalent. Other common autoimmune conditions include multiple sclerosis, ankylosing spondylitis, Graves' disease, rheumatoid arthritis, type 1 diabetes, lupus, Crohn's disease, ulcerated colitis, and celiac disease, among many others.

Autoimmune conditions tend to overlap—where one is present, there are often other autoimmune diseases lurking—and there is often a genetic component. However, it is important to note that different family members may have varying types of autoimmune disease. For example, in my extended family (parents, siblings, children, nieces, and nephews), one family member has ankylosing spondylitis, I have Hashimoto's and celiac disease (an autoimmune disease that occurs when ingesting gluten elicits an immune response that attacks the small intestine), and another family member has type 1 diabetes—all of which have stemmed from the same genetics but presented as different diseases.

While the mechanism and genetic links of autoimmune disease have been established, the exact cause remains unknown. According to the American Autoimmune-Related Diseases Association, autoimmune disease affects about 50 million Americans, nearly 16 percent of the population. The National Institutes of Health's numbers skew slightly lower, suggesting about 23.5 million Americans suffer from autoimmune disease. The difference in these numbers is based largely upon the illnesses the two organizations classify as autoimmune conditions, showing that this area of disease research is in need of further definition and clarification.

Current medical treatment for autoimmune disease focuses on immune system suppression (through medication, surgery, or radiation, among other ways), which can help stall the progress of the autoimmune disease but also affects the body's ability to fight off actual disease-causing organisms, lowering immunity to illness. However, many alternative therapies, such as dietary changes, are showing promise for helping people manage the symptoms associated with autoimmune disease.

Inflammation

Also part of the body's immune response is inflammation; without it, we can't get better. We are more acquainted with inflammation than we know. In fact, *itis* means inflammation, and any illness with the suffix *itis*—such as arthritis, colitis, laryngitis, bronchitis (inflammation of the joint, the colon, the larynx [voice box], and the lining of the bronchial tubes, respectively)—indicates inflammation.

When inflammation occurs, white blood cells are released into the blood or affected tissues to protect your body from unrecognized harmful substances. The surge of white blood cells increases blood flow to the target area and may result in redness and warmth. Some of the chemicals leak fluid into the tissues, which is what we know as swelling. Anyone who has ever had a bout of arthritis can attest to the painful effects of the inflammation response. In the case of Hashimoto's, the misdirected immune system can inflame the thyroid gland, further limiting its ability to produce critical hormones, and result in a goiter—an abnormal enlargement of the thyroid gland.

Because inflammation is so commonly present in autoimmune disorders, detecting its presence in blood tests often triggers physicians to perform further tests for autoimmune disease, although autoimmune diseases certainly aren't the only cause of inflammation. However, inflammation in the body can cause a host of symptoms that occur with autoimmune disease, such as pain, stiffness, fatigue, lethargy, swelling, fever, and similar symptoms. Therefore, managing inflammation (such as through dietary intervention) can, in many cases, help reduce signs and symptoms associated with autoimmune disease.

THE ROLE OF THE THYROID

It's hard to believe a small, butterfly-shaped gland at the front of your throat could cause you so much trouble, but believe it. The thyroid is a powerhouse in all it does for your body.

The Endocrine System

Your thyroid is an important part of your endocrine system—a grouping of hormone-producing glands that regulate growth and development, sexual function, tissue function, reproduction, metabolism, sleep, mood, and a host of other things. The endocrine system consists of the pituitary gland, thyroid gland, parathyroid glands, adrenal glands, pancreas, ovaries (in females), and testicles (in males). It is important to note that when it comes to regulating metabolism in the body, the thyroid is much more important than whether weight is packed on or melts off. *Every cell* in the body depends upon thyroid hormones for regulation of its metabolism (conversion of oxygen and calories to energy), so if the thyroid is having a bad day, it can affect the entire team of hormone functions. That's why people are often suffering from seemingly unrelated symptoms—the thyroid sets the rhythm of the system.

Thyroid Hormones

Your thyroid gland produces and distributes hormones that play a critical role in multiple functions throughout your body. The purpose of the thyroid gland is to take iodine, which is found in many foods, and convert it into thyroid hormones. Thyroid cells are the only cells in the body capable of absorbing iodine. These cells combine iodine and the amino acid tyrosine to produce three hormones:

Self-Compassion
The Best Investment You'll Ever Make

During this four-week plan, you may notice feelings of stress, anxiety, or fear arising. This is the time when it is most critical to practice self-compassion. Why? Treating yourself compassionately will help you stay calm, motivated, positive, clear, and strong as you adapt to new habits, gather information, and create new thought processes.

It's easy to be compassionate to others, but that harsh critic inside each of us is often much harder on us than it would ever be toward another person. And yet, you are worthy of compassion, especially from yourself. While it may feel self-indulgent, it is not. Instead, it is a deeply kind and caring act toward oneself, and it allows you to counteract your inner critic.

Self-compassion is kind and motivating. Instead of demoralizing you as your inner critic does, it lifts and supports you, just as you lift and support others when you offer them compassion. It is not justification for your actions or an attempt to make yourself feel better, but a way to care for yourself when you are feeling bad.

Benefits of self-compassion:

- Provides protection against anxiety and depression
- Promotes coping skills
- Increases self-motivation
- Improves emotional resilience
- Lowers stress
- Promotes inner joy and peace
- Allows you to practice compassion with others
- Quiets the inner critic
- Cultivates goodwill, allowing you to accept and be more at peace with your Hashimoto's diagnosis

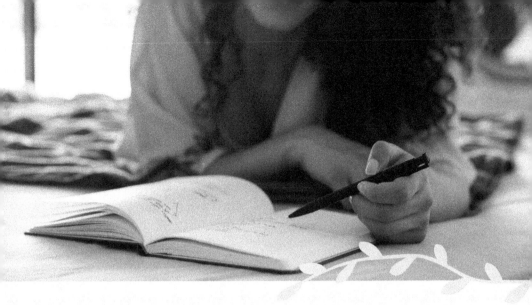

Try these three simple techniques for practicing self-compassion:

- Write a kind and gentle letter to yourself from the perspective of someone who loves you.
- Journal your feelings and then respond to any negativity as you would respond to a friend.
- When you observe your inner critic speaking to you harshly, take a one-minute self-compassion break. Close your eyes and place your hands gently over your heart. Breathe deeply and think, "May I treat myself with kindness."

Kristin Neff has written a wonderful book, *Self-Compassion: The Proven Power of Being Kind to Yourself,* from which this information was adapted, and which offers other suggestions for how to practice self-compassion. You can also find self-compassion exercises on her website, self-compassion.org.

We will discuss the critical nature of self-compassion in your Hashimoto's journey much more in chapter 4. For now, remember, in order to muster the power, will, and confidence within you to dedicate and commit to this four-week plan, you must believe in yourself and speak and treat yourself kindly, with more love and compassion.

- Triiodothyronine (T3, which contains three iodine molecules)
- Tetraiodothyronine (T4, or thyroxine, which contains four iodine molecules)
- Calcitonin (which helps maintain healthy levels of calcium in the blood and bones)

These hormones are then released into the blood stream and transported throughout the body to control metabolism.

According to the U.S. National Library of Medicine, the thyroid hormones T3 and T4 affect numerous body functions, including:

- Body temperature
- Metabolism (the process of converting fuel in food we eat into energy required to stimulate everything we do)
- Blood pressure
- Heart rate
- Clear thinking
- Nerve function
- Growth and brain maturation in children

Thyroid Function

When the level of thyroid hormones in your system is sluggish, it is detected first by the brain's hypothalamus, which tells the pituitary gland to give the thyroid a boost. A substance is released called, appropriately enough, thyroid-stimulating hormone (TSH). This hormone, in turn, stimulates the production of T3 and T4. So, three glands—thyroid, pituitary, and hypothalamus—work in concert to regulate the production and release of T3 and T4.

Thyroid Disease

Thyroid damage can occur in a number of ways. The most common forms of thyroid disease are:

- Hashimoto's thyroiditis (autoimmune hypothyroidism, or sluggish thyroid)
- Graves' disease (autoimmune hyperthyroidism, or overactive thyroid)
- Nonautoimmune hypothyroidism (mild thyroid failure)

The system can break down at any of the points along the way—from the hypothalamus to the thyroid. In the case of Hashimoto's thyroiditis, the breakdown occurs when your body thinks thyroid tissue is a foreign invader and begins to attack the healthy gland. As your immune system attacks your thyroid, damage occurs, and the gland begins to function abnormally. At first, the thyroid may show signs of hyperthyroidism, releasing excessive hormones, but as time passes, function slows and hormone production typically decreases. This results in the common symptoms you find associated with autoimmune and nonautoimmune hypothyroidism, such as poor body temperature control, fatigue, dry skin, hair loss, sluggishness, weight gain, and many other symptoms associated with poor metabolic regulation.

Causes

A number of factors can cause thyroid damage and disease, including:

- Poor diet
- Poor nutrient absorption (malabsorption)
- Environmental toxins
- Genetics
- Pituitary disorders
- Autoimmune disease
- Other hormonal disorders

Concurrent or Coexisting Conditions

People with autoimmune hypothyroidism may also experience other conditions or diseases that exist at the same time—known as "concurrent conditions." For example, I have the common cluster of Hashimoto's, celiac disease, and casein (milk protein) allergy. According to the National Institute of Diabetes and Digestive and Kidney Diseases, other conditions that often occur with Hashimoto's disease include:

- Vitiligo
- Rheumatoid arthritis
- Type 1 diabetes
- Addison's disease
- Pernicious anemia
- Celiac disease
- Autoimmune hepatitis

These concurrent conditions often make it difficult for health-care providers to diagnose Hashimoto's, because symptom clusters for multiple conditions muddy the water and confuse doctors and patients alike. For instance, many of my celiac disease symptoms are not consistent with symptoms common in Hashimoto's thyroiditis, so as I related my symptoms to my doctors, they were unable to match all of them with one specific condition.

COMMON CAUSES OF HASHIMOTO'S THYROIDITIS

Hashimoto's thyroiditis is one form of autoimmune thyroid disease (the other is Graves' disease). Autoimmune diseases, including Hashimoto's disease, have been on the rise throughout the developed world in the past decades, according to a June 2012 report in *Medical News Today*. This suggests environmental factors may be at play in the development of diseases like Hashimoto's, but research is still ongoing. However, as autoimmune conditions abound, one can't help but wonder about toxins in our environment, the standard Western diet full of artificial and processed foods, stress, and other manmade issues, as possible causes.

There is some evidence that genetics contribute to developing Hashimoto's disease. According to an article in the 2005 *Journal of Autoimmune Diseases*, Hashimoto's has a strong genetic component. Therefore, if someone in your family has Hashimoto's disease, you have a stronger predisposition to develop it, or another autoimmune disease, yourself.

Triggers

If you have a genetic disposition to Hashimoto's (or any other autoimmune disease), it doesn't mean you will develop the illness. In most cases, other factors must exist that trigger the gene, leading to the onset of disease. Here are some of the triggers: ·

Iodine

As previously noted, iodine is a key component of the thyroid hormones T3 and T4. Therefore, iodine plays a key role in developing autoimmune thyroid disease, but it may not be as straightforward as iodine = good, lack of iodine = bad. In fact, studies have shown the relationship between iodine and thyroid disease to be a complex one, so drop the salt shaker!

However, there are contradictions in the importance of iodine to thyroid health. An article in the December 1998 issue of the journal *Thyroid*, "The Epidemiology of Thyroid Disease in Iodine Sufficiency," and another article in the June 2011 issue of the *British Medical Bulletin*, "The Epidemiology of Thyroid Disease," highlight the contradictions of the iodine-thyroid relationship.

From the *British Medical Bulletin*:

- The manifestation of thyroid disease is determined by iodine availability.
- Worldwide iodine deficiency is a common cause of thyroid disorders.

From *Thyroid*:

- Autoimmune thyroid disease is much more common in areas of iodine sufficiency than in areas of iodine deficiency.
- The incidence of autoimmune hyperthyroidism increases upward for up to four years in areas after iodine is added to table salt.

These appear to be two very disparate sets of findings. Clearly, there is a correlation between iodine and autoimmune thyroidism, but what is it? Functional medicine specialist Chris Kresser offers a potential explanation, noting iodine intake, especially in supplemental form, can increase the autoimmune attack on the thyroid. However, Kresser also notes supplemental iodine may bring about cases of autoimmune thyroid disease only when the mineral selenium (found in tuna and Brazil nuts, for instance) is deficient. That's because selenium *appears* to be protective against potential toxic effects of iodine as it relates to autoimmune hypothyroidism. Therefore, a combination of the two, preferably from dietary sources, not supplementary sources like table salt, appears to be helpful in fighting Hashimoto's thyroiditis.

Since both supplemental iodine and supplemental selenium can be dangerous in high doses, it is best to try to derive both from food sources. If you do feel you may need to supplement either of these nutrients, it is important to work closely with your doctor to avoid toxicity or unintended consequences.

Being Female

Hey, ladies, lucky us! We are seven times more likely to develop Hashimoto's than men, according to a WomensHealth.gov Hashimoto's disease fact sheet. While it can occur at any age (mine presented when I was twenty-two), it most commonly occurs in middle age.

Pregnancy and Perimenopause

A woman's estrogen and hormone levels fluctuate wildly during these two times of life. This can trigger inflammation and the expression of Hashimoto's in women who are genetically susceptible, according to functional medicine specialist Chris Kresser.

Other Autoimmune Diseases

As previously mentioned, other autoimmune diseases can trigger the onset of Hashimoto's disease. These illnesses frequently occur in clusters, although it's difficult to know whether the other diseases triggered Hashimoto's or vice versa.

Leaky Gut

If you've done any research into autoimmune diseases, you've probably come across the term "leaky gut syndrome." According to an article in the February 2013 issue of *Today's Dietician*, leaky gut (also known as intestinal permeability) may be a factor.

Leaky gut syndrome goes a little something like this: The standard Western diet (along with other environmental factors) is high in toxic substances that cause damage to junctions in the intestines. When this damage occurs, the intestines become permeable, and molecules of undigested food leak out into the bloodstream. This overstimulates the immune system, which goes on full foreign-invader alert and begins to attack healthy tissue. Bam! Autoimmune disease, such as Hashimoto's thyroiditis, develops.

Small Intestinal Bacterial Overgrowth (SIBO)

Today's Dietician also cites SIBO as a potential cause of autoimmune diseases such as Hashimoto's. As the name implies, SIBO is an overgrowth of bacteria in the intestine. While research is ongoing, several risk factors for the overgrowth of bacteria have been identified, including:

- Decreased gut motility (poor contraction of intestinal muscles)
- Surgery
- Diverticulitis
- Gluten intolerance and celiac disease
- Other malabsorption syndromes
- Pancreatic inflammation
- Certain medications such as proton pump inhibitors (Nexium, Prilosec, and others)

Other Potential Triggers

There are many other possible common factors for Hashimoto's disease. While one of these items may or may not trigger it on its own, in combination with multiple triggers, the potential for developing Hashimoto's may increase. These include:

- Sensitivity to gluten
- Excessive ingestion of goitrogenic foods (such as soy and the cruciferous vegetables, including broccoli, cabbage, kale, and cauliflower)
- Sensitivity to nightshades, a family of flowering plants that includes several popular crops (like tomatoes and eggplant), medicinal plants, spices, weeds, and ornamentals
- Sensitivity to dairy products

- Other food sensitivities
- Low iron
- Low vitamin D
- Other nutritional deficiencies
- Poor blood sugar control
- Candida
- Chronic stress
- Poorly functioning adrenals
- Hormone imbalance
- Chemicals and toxins in the diet and environment
- Certain medications

While these factors are frequently debated and research is ongoing, these are commonly listed threats for Hashimoto's, and many may have merit. For example, I saw the biggest flare-up of my symptoms when I was on a vegan diet and eating a lot of soy, which is a goitrogenic food. While this is an anecdotal piece of evidence, eliminating soy helped, and there isn't currently any scientific proof for or against this theory. This is the case for many of the above-listed factors, which also have anecdotal but not scientific evidence suggesting they may play a role. Many of these issues and imbalances will be covered in the diet section of this book, while others will be addressed with lifestyle modifications.

CHAPTER 1 TO-DOS

☐ Share your plans to begin this four-week program and ask the support of friends, family, and coworkers.

☐ Make it a priority to be more in tune with, and aware of, your body and mind. Monitoring changes in your normal behaviors and feelings is critical when tracking what kinds of shifts—dietary, lifestyle, emotional—could benefit you, as well as determining what changes are actually effective.

☐ Begin the process of self-care by setting aside a few minutes every day to do something for yourself, whether it's an exercise class, meditation, or eating a good meal.

☐ Make "no" part of your vocabulary by identifying and eliminating some busywork that adds unnecessary stress to your life.

☐ Join an online Hashimoto's community, or check out a site like stopthethyroidmadness.com, to share with others who may have similar experiences and helpful advice. Sharing information, or just knowing others out there "get you," can make all the difference, especially on those bad days when you need help keeping your chin up.

DAILY CHECK-IN

Pausing to check in with your body is helpful in tracking your health.

☐ Scan your body and notice any physical sensations.

☐ Turn your attention inward and notice any thoughts or feelings that come up.

☐ Remember that changes to your diet, stress levels, or rest can affect how you're feeling right now.

☐ Do something nice for yourself to cultivate feelings of well-being.

2

HASHIMOTO'S THYROIDITIS: A CHRONIC CONDITION

Hashimoto's disease is one of dozens of "invisible illnesses"—those illnesses that you can feel intensely but others most likely cannot see because you don't "look sick." Hashimoto's manifests differently in different people at different times. In the beginning, you may have days when you feel fantastic, and others when you can barely get off the couch. Because Hashimoto's symptoms are mind-body integrated, it's difficult to accept them as an actual physical illness instead of a mental one. I often found myself wondering if it was all in my head.

After living with this condition, and other autoimmune disease, for 25 years I can tell you this: It's not all in your head. You have a chronic and frustrating condition, and what you are experiencing are physical manifestations of an invisible illness.

STUCK IN A STATE OF CHRONIC DYSFUNCTION

Your body, specifically your immune system, has declared war on your thyroid gland. Like a good soldier going to battle, your immune system is relentless, continuously attacking its enemy and destroying it bit by bit. Unfortunately, your immune system has identified the wrong enemy. It is performing its nonstop raids against an innocent party, and the casualties of this war are your health and well-being.

Hashimoto's is a progressive autoimmune disease, which is a fancy way of saying that over time and without treatment the condition worsens, grows, or spreads. As your immune system launches an attack on your thyroid, the gland begins to function less. As the attack continues, your thyroid will produce fewer thyroid hormones as time goes on. In the beginning, you may feel sluggish on some days as thyroid hormones are reduced, and completely fine on other days, when your hormones are less affected. If your doctor catches the illness early and provides medication, you may even experience "hyper" days due to your medication providing more hormones than your body needs, only for your thyroid to start underproducing again. This was a pattern I experienced during the early days of my illness: I had good days and bad days, until after a time, the good days became outnumbered by bad days.

As the disease progresses and more of your thyroid is destroyed, you slip into a state of chronic hormone underproduction known as hypothyroidism (underactive thyroid). During this stage, you may begin to experience:

- Fatigue
- Lethargy
- Sensitivity to cold (I was cold all the time!)
- Muscle and joint aches and pains
- Constipation
- Brain fog
- Weight gain or difficulty losing weight
- Slowed metabolism

- Hoarsening or deepening of the voice
- A strangling or tight sensation in the throat
- Heavy or prolonged menstruation
- Dry skin
- Enlarged thyroid (goiter)

Fluctuating TSH

One of the frustrations associated with Hashimoto's is difficulty obtaining a diagnosis. Part of the reason this occurs is fluctuating TSH (thyroid-stimulating hormone) levels. One test may show normal TSH ranges, while others may show elevated or even lowered TSH. There's a reason for this.

If you recall in chapter 1 (see page 22), I described how the pituitary gland releases TSH in response to the amount of T3 and T4 present in the blood. When T3 and T4 levels are low, the pituitary gland releases more TSH to stimulate production of the hormones. When the levels are high, the pituitary gland releases less TSH in order to level out thyroid hormones. In the case of Hashimoto's, particularly in the early stages, fluctuating levels of thyroid hormone in your blood will lead to fluctuating levels of TSH.

Untreated Hashimoto's

If your illness goes undiagnosed and untreated as mine did for more than 20 years, you get caught up in a cycle of illness. As your thyroid slowly dies under its constant assault from your immune system, you eventually become fully hypothyroid, and your body greatly slows its production of thyroid hormones. As time passes, your symptoms worsen. The Mayo Clinic notes that untreated Hashimoto's can cause a host of problems, including:

- Large goiter that affects breathing and swallowing
- Heart problems and heart failure
- High cholesterol
- High blood pressure
- Loss of libido
- Depression
- A life-threatening condition called myxedema (swelling of the skin and underlying tissue)

A June 25, 2013, *New York Times* Health Guide called "Chronic Thyroiditis (Hashimoto's Disease)" notes that other conditions can occur with untreated Hashimoto's, including:

- Anemia
- Respiratory issues
- Impaired kidney function
- Headaches
- Glaucoma
- Decreased fertility

Difficulty with Diagnosis

Along with fluctuating TSH levels, Hashimoto's can defy diagnosis for a number of other reasons.

Concurrent Conditions

Symptoms associated with concurrent conditions can make diagnosing Hashimoto's far more difficult. For example, in my case I also had undiagnosed celiac disease, which presented with symptoms not typically associated with Hashimoto's like diarrhea, gas, bloating, cramping, and multiple issues associated with nutrient malabsorption.

Progression of Symptoms

Because Hashimoto's is a progressive disease, the symptoms change over time. This can make diagnosing it more difficult as symptoms change.

Complications

Complications of Hashimoto's, such as poor sleep, insulin resistance, and weight gain, may present with their own symptoms that disguise those of Hashimoto's. I can attest to this, as for years most of my healthcare providers diagnosed me with obesity and told me every single symptom I had was related to the numbers on the scale (see My Misdiagnosis Nightmare on page 38).

Diagnosing the Condition

As my 20-plus-year journey to diagnosis suggests, obtaining a diagnosis of Hashimoto's can be tricky. A person suffering from Hashimoto's can have multiple negative tests, which earlier or later could turn out to be positive. Others may feel well but have abnormal antibody test results, meaning antibodies are present and possibly lurking to attack your healthy thyroid.

The first step in obtaining a diagnosis is paying close attention to your symptoms. I highly recommend tracking all your symptoms with the Daily Checklists provided at the end of each chapter—even those you think might be no big deal or embarrass you. For example, in the first few years I sought diagnosis, I had recurring mental-emotional symptoms that were highly unusual for me, but I wrote them off for two reasons:

1. I was in denial that they were symptoms at all.

2. I was slightly (or greatly) concerned that such symptoms would lead to a diagnosis of mental illness.

I am fully convinced this is part of the reason my diagnosis was missed in the early years. I failed to record and report all my symptoms, so by the time I realized they were symptoms and was ready to discuss them, I'd gained so much weight that obesity became the prevailing diagnosis.

Learn from my mistake. Record your symptoms over days and weeks. Record them all, and report them to your healthcare provider as you seek diagnosis.

Of course, symptom reporting is just the first step in obtaining diagnosis. Your healthcare provider will also want to perform a thorough physical examination, and may order blood tests. Since it's your job to advocate for yourself, it's perfectly fine to ask for specific tests if you suspect Hashimoto's thyroiditis.

Advocating for Yourself about Labs

The following tests may be helpful in obtaining diagnosis, but keep in mind that if your tests come back normal, it doesn't necessarily mean you don't have Hashimoto's. Tests can confirm but not exclude a diagnosis. Due to the nature of fluctuating hormones, including T3, T4, and TSH, negative results happen, even though they may later be positive.

When I first started seeking diagnosis, the doctors ʼ
only testing my TSH. In fact, for the first several years ⌐
diagnosis, I thought TSH was the only test for hypothyroidıs.
It wasn't until I started talking with other people experiencing
problems similar to mine that I discovered other tests were available that could also diagnose hypothyroidism and Hashimoto's.
Through these interactions with others, I also discovered many
others faced a similar problem in their doctor's offices.

It's important to understand that just because your TSH test
is "normal," it doesn't mean your thyroid is normal. Request that
your doctor also conduct T4 and T3 tests, as well as TPO and Tg
antibody tests to look for autoimmune hypothyroidism. Once
diagnosed, it may also be beneficial to ask your doctor to perform
the antibody test every six to twelve months in order to determine
how effectively your treatment plan is working, or even if you have
entered remission.

You are the keeper of your health, so tracking how you feel
and speaking up in the doctor's office is essential in helping you
achieve your best health.

Thyroid-Specific Tests

You and your provider may wish to review the following tests.
Here's what each test looks for, and what the results may indicate:

- **TSH:** This is a blood test. There are two types of TSH tests:
  normal TSH and sensitive TSH. It's important to request the
  sensitive TSH test, which is, you guessed it, more sensitive.
  The sensitive TSH requires morning fasting, while regular
  TSH does not. Higher levels of TSH in the bloodstream indicate
  lower levels of thyroid hormones. A normal range for TSH is
  between 0.4 and 4.2.

- **Total T4 (TT4):** This blood test measures the total amount
  of T4 in your bloodstream. Low levels may indicate insufficient
  T4 production or insufficient levels of TSH. A normal range for
  TT4 is 4.5 to 11.5.

- **Total T3 (TT3):** This blood test measures the total amount of T3 in your bloodstream. Low levels of T3 may indicate poor thyroid function, while high levels indicate hyperthyroidism. A normal range for TT3 is 75 to 200.

- **Free T3 (FT3):** This blood test measures T3 molecules that are not bound to protein in the bloodstream. While it is most helpful in diagnosing hyperthyroidism, it may also give your doctor a better picture of your overall thyroid health. A normal range for FT3 is 260 to 480 pg/dL or 4 to 7.4 pmol/L.

- **Free T4 (FT4):** This blood test measures T4 that isn't bound to protein in the bloodstream. A normal range is 0.7 to 2.0.

- **Thyroid peroxidase (TPO) antibodies:** The presence of TPO antibodies in your bloodstream may indicate the presence of an autoimmune source for thyroid disease, although their absence doesn't necessarily mean autoimmune disease is not present. Therefore, this blood test can only confirm autoimmune disease, not exclude it.

- **Thyroglobulin (Tg) antibodies:** This blood test measures another type of antibody that may be present in autoimmune thyroid disease. A negative test means no antibodies are present, but it doesn't rule out autoimmune disease; however, the presence of the antibodies may confirm the disease.

- **TRH test:** This blood test checks to make sure the hypothalamus and pituitary glands are working correctly and in concert with the thyroid triad (hypothalamus, pituitary, and thyroid).

Tests for Concurrent Conditions

If you suspect you may have concurrent conditions, like I do, you may wish to request other tests:

- **C-reactive protein (CRP):** This blood test may indicate inflammation, which is present in autoimmune disease.

- **Complete blood count (CBC):** This measures red and white cells in your blood, which can indicate infection or elevated white cells, which may be present in autoimmune disease.

- **Autoantibody tests:** These can suggest whether autoimmune disease is present by detecting the presence of antibodies.
- **tTG-IgA test:** This test looks for antibodies specific to celiac disease, but it will be positive only if you are eating gluten in your diet.

If you suspect other conditions, discuss further testing with your doctor to help you obtain an accurate diagnosis.

The Mask of Mental Illness

An important culprit in your diagnosis pursuit is the uncanny similarities between thyroiditis and mental illness. According to the Thyroid Foundation of Canada, the psychiatric disturbances of both hyperthyroidism and hypothyroidism mimic mental illness. For instance, those with overactive thyroid may exhibit marked anxiety and tension, emotional mood swings, impatience and irritability, compulsive overactivity, oversensitivity to noise, bouts of depression with sadness, and problems with sleep and appetite. An underactive thyroid can lead to mounting loss of interest and ambition or drive, brain fog, lack of concentration, poor short-term memory, change in personality and liveliness, general intellectual deterioration, depression with a touch of paranoia, and eventually, if not checked, dementia and permanent harmful effects on the brain. In instances of each condition, people have been misdiagnosed, hospitalized for months, and treated without success for psychosis.

To feel as if you are going crazy and to have people suggest you need an antidepressant or antianxiety medication can add to the already burgeoning stress of your medical mystery, which can further perpetuate the thyroid dysfunction cycle. Seek treatment for your emotional symptoms, and be sure to mention to your doctor or therapist that you would like your thyroid tested as well. Do not be embarrassed about sharing what you are feeling, no matter how irrational, hopeless, or impulsive. So many people suffer from both thyroiditis and mental issues, and there is nothing shameful about either! You deserve to feel good, and you can, by providing empathy, compassion, and advocacy to yourself.

My Misdiagnosis Nightmare

I n my 20s, I was healthy and active, working as a fitness trainer. One night I went to bed healthy, the next morning I woke up sick. My health was never the same.

Within five or six months' time, I gained about 80 pounds. I started experiencing debilitating exhaustion, severe muscle pain, anxiety, and mood swings. I shared my physical symptoms with doctors but hid the mental symptoms of anxiety, fearful of what those symptoms might mean. I wish I hadn't. Talking about my mental symptoms could have helped lead to a quicker diagnosis.

Doctors told me that in order to get better, I needed to lose weight. I grew frustrated because I was still working as a fitness instructor and eating only 1,200 to 1,500 calories per day, yet the weight piled on.

Occasionally, doctors would test my TSH levels, which looked normal, so no one was willing to look further. Doctors couldn't find a discernible pattern with my tests, and due to symptoms from undiagnosed concurrent conditions, I didn't present in a way that resembled a thyroid condition.

I continued to gain weight and suffer symptoms. While doctors told me to eat less and move more, my attempts to exercise left me sicker. Eventually, exhaustion and pain kept me from the gym, and my quality of life deteriorated.

In 2009, a nurse practitioner recognized my cluster of symptoms as Hashimoto's and ordered an array of tests. I believe she deduced that the problem stemmed from my thyroid because she questioned me about my mental issues. This time, I was honest about them.

Treating the Hashimoto's with thyroid medications helped lessen some of the symptoms, particularly those related to mood, but weight loss remained a challenge, and many of my physical symptoms lingered. Likewise, persistent gut symptoms remained, which later led to tests diagnosing celiac disease and casein allergy. Those concurrent diseases became the final piece of the puzzle. Once I changed my diet (while still taking medication), I finally was able to return to better health. Today, as long as I am careful about what I eat, I feel healthy and energetic. I've also lost 125 pounds and am back to my sunny, even-tempered self.

If I hadn't educated myself, advocated persistently, and detailed my mental and physical symptoms, I might still be sick and getting progressively worse. That's why it's important to report all symptoms to your doctor, as well as educate and advocate for yourself on your journey to better health.

TREATMENT OPTIONS

As I sought diagnosis and treatment for my Hashimoto's, I had a single goal in mind: to get my life back. Many people with Hashimoto's have the same goal, although what this means is highly personal. For me, it meant returning to a state where illness, pain, and exhaustion didn't rule my life anymore, and being able to engage in life in an active and meaningful way. For you, it may mean something else. However, in general, the goal with Hashimoto's treatment is to help forestall the progression of the disease, restore normal bodily functions, and minimize symptoms.

It's important to note that the damage to your thyroid from the autoimmune attacks is irreversible, and it is unlikely your body will ever restore the tissue damage to your thyroid. With less thyroid tissue, your body will continue to struggle to make adequate thyroid hormones. Therefore, chances are, you may require the use of replacement thyroid hormones, and always will. This is why medication is one important intervention for people with Hashimoto's thyroiditis. Other interventions focus on lifestyle and diet in an attempt to slow or halt the immune system's destruction of the thyroid.

Medication

Thyroid medication serves as hormone replacement, putting back in the thyroid hormones your body either underproduces or has stopped making altogether. The type and amount of hormone replacement may vary throughout your life, based on various factors. For instance, if the damage to your thyroid progresses, the amount of hormones your body produces will likely lower. This could lead to the need for increasing your hormone dosage. Likewise, changes in diet, activity levels, concurrent conditions, issues like malabsorption or low stomach acid, body weight changes, medications, and other factors may increase or reduce your required dosage.

I was on a dose of 4.5 grains of my natural desiccated thyroid medication when I started losing weight. After I had lost about 50 pounds, I started to notice my heart racing, particularly at night, and I was having difficulty sleeping and felt generally edgy. Blood tests revealed I was hyperthyroid, indicating I needed to reduce the dosage of my thyroid medications. We stepped down by 1.5 grains until my symptoms and hormone ranges normalized. This is an example of why it is important to continue to monitor your symptoms and the levels of thyroid hormones in your blood. Your close attention to symptoms and a strong partnership with your doctor are essential in this process.

Types of Medication

While it seems like a basic idea, there is actually quite a bit of controversy about the type of thyroid medications people with Hashimoto's should take. Some people swear by natural desiccated thyroid (NDT) medication, which typically comes from porcine (pig) or bovine (cow) sources. Others, including many doctors, believe NDT contains poorly regulated doses of thyroid hormone and are therefore inferior to synthetic (laboratory-made) hormones.

Both sides of the issue have valid points, and I know people who have better results with different types. I have taken both NDT and synthetic hormones and discovered that, *for me,* NDT offers better symptom relief. However, that doesn't necessarily mean it will work best for you. Although I've said it many times, I need to reiterate it here: Partnership with your doctor and active participation in your treatment is vital in your Hashimoto's journey. Because it's up to you, in close partnership with your doctor, to find the medication solution that works best for you.

The common types of thyroid medication include:

- **Natural desiccated thyroid (NDT):** This is thyroid derived from animal (typically pig) thyroids. I take one type of this medication, Armour Thyroid, which I call "every part of the pig including the thyroid." The first time I opened my pill bottle, I swore I detected a faint whiff of bacon. NDT contains both T3 and T4 and is the only thyroid medication that contains both hormones. Vegetarians and people with dietary restrictions prohibiting pork may not be comfortable with this medication.

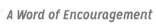 *A Word of Encouragement*

Your mind and spirit are just as important as your body is in your health journey. Use visualization to improve your health. Take a quiet moment each day to picture yourself in vibrant good health, allowing your thoughts and beliefs about yourself to manifest in your life.

Not all NDT is the same. While all NDT comes from animal sources and contains similar types and amounts of hormones, the binders and fillers in the pills may vary. Likewise, the manufacturer may change the ingredients without notice from time to time. Back in about 2009, I noticed my Armour Thyroid seemed to stop working as well. I had just renewed my prescription and almost overnight I noticed a return of some of my symptoms. At the time, I also participated in a community of other Hashimoto's sufferers, and several other people were noticing the same thing. After some research, I discovered that the manufacturer had changed the binding in the pills to cellulose, and I suspected the cellulose binding might be affecting absorption of the medication. At someone else's suggestion, I started crushing the pills and taking them under my tongue. My symptoms disappeared again. The moral of the story is: small changes may alter how your medication works. Monitor your symptoms and work closely with your doctor!

- *Levothyroxine:* This is a synthetic T4-only medication. Your body converts the T4 in the medication to T3 as needed. This is the most frequently prescribed form of thyroid medication. One example of levothyroxine is Synthroid.

- *Synthetic T3:* Some doctors prefer to prescribe a synthetic T3 like Cytomel alone or in combination with levothyroxine. Your body uses T3 very quickly, so dosing may be an issue for some people. To remedy this, many doctors recommend split dosing, or taking the medication twice a day.

Generic versus Name Brand Medications

Pharmacists will tell you that the generic versions of medication have the exact same efficacy and function as name brands like Synthroid. In truth, a number of factors that go into the manufacture of the medication may change how it functions in your body; often differences are highly individual.

For example, I previously mentioned that when I was taking Armour Thyroid medication, it suddenly stopped working for me because the manufacturer changed the binding they used. There are similar differences between generic and name brand meds, so it's important to work with your doctor to find the medication that works best for you—and this can be highly individual. Be willing to try a new type of medication if yours isn't working. For example, if you're taking a generic T4 medication and not seeing results, ask your doctor to switch you to Synthroid, etc.

Taking the Meds

Most doctors recommend taking thyroid medication on an empty stomach, first thing in the morning, and then waiting an hour to eat.

Some supplements and medications—iron, calcium, and antacids—can block the absorption of thyroid medication. Therefore, it is recommended you space dosing by at least two hours to ensure your body fully absorbs the medication.

Because of this potential to inhibit absorption of thyroid meds, it is important your doctor has a complete list of all medications and supplements you take. To avoid possible interactions, I take my thyroid medication first thing in the morning (usually about six o'clock). Since iron and calcium can also block each other, I take my iron in the mid-afternoon at around two o'clock, and then take my calcium in the evening at about eight o'clock. With some thought, you can find a schedule that works for you.

Lifestyle Modifications

Some healthcare providers, particularly alternative practitioners, suggest lifestyle and dietary modifications to help with Hashimoto's, in addition to medication. These lifestyle and dietary modifications may have several different goals, including:

- Managing symptoms
- Minimizing or halting damage to the thyroid
- Minimizing or eliminating inflammation
- Decreasing factors that may contribute to symptoms and/or autoimmune disease such as chemicals, toxins, stress, poor sleep, and other elements

I discuss and recommend many of these lifestyle modifications throughout this book. It's important that you determine which will be of value to you, because not every remedy works for every person, since your body and its needs are unique. It's up to you to experiment and listen to your own internal wisdom.

YOUR HASHIMOTO'S HEALTH TEAM

While many people look at their doctor as the absolute authority when it comes to their health, I think it's important you be an even more active participant in your healthcare than any of your doctors. As a health expert, your doctor serves in an advisory capacity, but *you* are the only expert on you. Your relationship with all members of your Hashimoto's healthcare team should be a very active and collaborative one, with you at the helm of the operation.

Your doctors can only respond to information you provide them, along with any information gleaned from examination and testing. However, if you don't clearly or accurately report your symptoms, your doctor may not know what to test for. This is why your role on your healthcare team is the most important one: You are the only one who lives in your body and knows how you feel. It's up to you to be your best advocate, sharing when treatments don't work, asking for more help if you need it, and continuing to gently insist on accurate diagnoses and compassionate treatment. Good doctors will not only welcome your active role in your care, they will demand it.

It's important to find healthcare providers who:

- Listen to what you have to say and respond to your questions or concerns

- Discuss diagnosis and treatment with you in a way you understand
- Allow and encourage you to be an active partner in your care
- Display willingness to work with others on your integrated team, if you have built one

You may choose many team members or a single provider. It's all a matter of your condition(s) and what works best for you. Some team members to consider include:

- *Primary care provider (PCP):* This is your main healthcare provider, the one who has the big picture of your health. While your PCP may refer you to other doctors, he or she is the anchor. For your PCP, you might choose an internist, a family practitioner, or a nurse practitioner, among others. My PCP is a medical doctor who is also a functional medicine specialist focused on overall health via diet and lifestyle.

- *Endocrinologist:* An endocrinologist specializes in diagnosis and treatment of endocrine disorders (thyroid disorder is an endocrine disease). While not everyone needs an endocrinologist, some people with Hashimoto's probably need one, including pregnant women, women trying to become pregnant, babies, and children. If you have a difficult-to-diagnose endocrine illness, multiple thyroid disorders, goiter, or other conditions like heart disease, it is probably best to seek one.

- *Nutrition specialist:* While this isn't strictly necessary, working with a nutrition specialist may be helpful, in addition to your medical team. Nutrition experts can help you assess your own dietary needs, address supplementation issues, and more. You have multiple options for this type of healthcare provider, including naturopathic doctors, functional medicine specialists, registered dieticians, and nutritionists.

- *Other specialists:* You may have other healthcare needs relating to coexisting conditions. Your PCP can help you with referrals to the right types of healthcare providers such as gastroenterologists, neurologists, dermatologists, and others.

- *Additional self-care providers:* Other practitioners on my team include a massage therapist, a chiropractor, an aromatherapist, and an energy healer. While these aren't necessary, they play an important role in my health and well-being, plus I look forward to my visits as part of my "me time" necessary for my self-care.

The Impact of Hashimoto's on Relationships

As someone who has had Hashimoto's for most of my adult life, I feel truly qualified to write about its impact on my relationships. I'd like to be able to assure you that Hashimoto's doesn't affect relationships, but the truth is, it does. When you are chronically ill, you may find you have to say no to people more often than you wish. I know this was true for me for many years. Likewise, some people have difficulty understanding chronic "invisible" illness, because they can't *see* your limitations. In intimate partnership relationships, issues like loss of energy or lack of libido may take a toll. In some cases, this may render relationships more difficult and tense, or even cause them to end. However, there are some steps you can take to help you maintain and build relationships of all kinds:

- Explain your Hashimoto's from a medical and technical standpoint and how it manifests, and set realistic expectations about how you can participate in relationships.
- Learn to say no nicely.
- Allow others to help you if they offer. While it may feel humbling to accept help, it is actually a gift you are giving to others in allowing them to feel helpful and supportive.
- Don't be afraid to state your needs and ask what other people need from you. Then, negotiate a solution that works well for you both.
- Don't say yes when you mean no, because it can build resentment.

RECOGNIZING WHAT WORKS AND WHAT DOESN'T

When you're chronically ill, you receive lots of advice from well-meaning people. Everyone has the newest thing they heard about, or that worked for their great-aunt's best friend's neighbor, and they just know it will work for you. Some of this information may be valid; others, not so much. I have probably heard thousands of pieces of advice over the years. Some of it sounded intriguing, and some of it sounded, quite frankly, nuts.

So how do you know what to try, and how do you know if it works? This is where your inner wisdom comes in quite handy.

Filter

Before you try anything, take a moment to consider:

- **The source:** Does it come from a credible source, such as a physician or an expert in the field, or does it come fourth- or fifth-hand from somebody who heard about somebody, who heard about somebody?

- **Scientific evidence:** What do credible health and medical sources say about it? Have there been any studies done? What do the studies say?

- **Anecdotal evidence:** While anecdotal evidence doesn't meet the same stringent standards as scientific studies, there is still value in the experience of others. Do your research and see what others are saying. Don't look at just one person's experience; look at experiences described by a variety of people.

- **Lifestyle compatibility:** Will the change fit within your lifestyle? Can you afford it? Do you have the time? Do you have the motivation?

- **Logic:** Does it make logical sense to you, or does it sound like a stretch? Can you see how the intervention might actually lead to the claimed results?

- **Trustworthiness:** Is it snake oil? There are plenty of unscrupulous people waiting to capitalize and profit off your desire to feel better. Beware of quick fixes and products that seem too good to be true (and that require a credit card number).
- **Your biology:** Your biology is unique and might not respond to the same remedies as someone else's. I understand the disappointment that arises when something that sounded really promising doesn't work, but it doesn't make things hopeless. It just means you need to find those interventions and lifestyle modifications that provide you benefit, because your body isn't exactly like everyone else's.

Consult

It's always important to work in partnership with your healthcare providers. Before starting any treatment or lifestyle intervention, make sure that it isn't contraindicated with your condition or medications, and that it isn't something that could be dangerous to your health.

Try

Once you've arrived at something you'd like to try, do it. Try only one intervention at a time. Commit to a period of two to four weeks of strict adherence to the intervention/lifestyle change to see how it works to you. Before you start, spend a week recording your symptoms. Then, track your symptoms daily throughout the intervention, comparing them to how you felt previously.

Tune In

Listen carefully to your body; it will tell you whether the intervention is working. Does it make you feel better, either physically or mentally/emotionally? If you see improvement, it's up to you to determine whether the improvements are enough to continue, or whether it's time to let the intervention go.

Gently Speak Up for Yourself
and Your Needs

....

During the course of the next four weeks, you're going to need to set aside time for yourself, ideally an hour a day, or as much as you can. This important time avoids all frivolous undertakings and outside demands and responsibilities. If this isn't something you've regularly done in the past, it may be difficult to kindly assert yourself.

I was not always adept at speaking up for my needs, especially in the beginning. I often found myself apologizing after I explained it was "me time." Over the years, however, I have learned how to exude quiet strength and self-possession, gently asserting myself in order to have my own needs met. And I no longer feel guilty or bad about it.

The first and most important step in gentle self-assertion is knowing, under-standing, and believing what you are asking for is necessary and deserved. You must know deep inside that what you need is important for your health and well-being. And, in turn, when your needs are being met, you are also better able to meet the needs of your loved ones. Therefore, you must attend to your own well-being to be at your best in every relationship, whether it is with family, friends, or even healthcare providers.

Once you trust that your needs are vital to your self-care and the care of others, it is easier to advocate for yourself in every relationship.

Some tips for kind self-assertion:

- Set the stage by explaining what you are doing and why, and sharing how you may need to put aside some tasks in order to really focus on getting well, not just for your sake, but for the sake of everyone around you.
- Ask for support from your loved ones, making them partners in your health and well-being.
- Whenever possible, communicate your needs ahead of time. For example, the night before an activity, you might tell your spouse and children that tomorrow at a certain time you will be unavailable, because you are doing something to support your health.

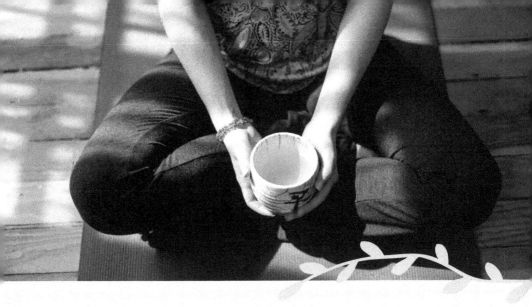

- Make "no" part of your vocabulary. It can be said nicely, "No, thank you," but it doesn't require justification or explanation. Simply say no. If you are asked again, smile and say no again. Doing this is empowering, and it gets easier as you go along.
- Communicate your needs using "I" messages, especially if you have a difficult message to deliver. Use the formula, "When you . . . I feel. . . ." For example, "When you don't help me clean up after dinner, I feel frustrated and anxious."
- When someone has helped you in a way that supports your health, tell them. Positive feedback goes a long way. For instance, "When you did the dishes last night, my 10 minutes on the couch really helped me reboot."
- Check out the book *Nonviolent Communication: A Language of Life* by Marshall B. Rosenberg, PhD, for plenty of techniques for gently communicating with others.

Track

Tracking symptoms—not just physical, but mental and emotional—
is essential. Track symptoms throughout the process (before,
during, and after). Get in the habit of doing a daily check-in,
like the one that appears at the end of each chapter in part 1.
Analyze this data.

- If you feel worse during the intervention, stop. Do the symptoms go away when you stop? If so, the intervention may be
  more harmful than helpful. If the symptoms continue, then
  they may be unassociated with the intervention.

- In some cases, recovery symptoms may occur. These symptoms tend to be mild to moderate and arise in the first days
  or week of an intervention as the body responds to the intervention. If you continue, and the symptoms dissipate after
  a week and don't recur, then you probably were experiencing
  recovery symptoms.

- Always stop an intervention when there are severe symptoms,
  and talk with your doctor.

- If you have new symptoms, stop the intervention and see
  if they go away. If they do, chances are they were related to
  the intervention.

- If your symptoms improve during the intervention, then it's
  up to you to determine how much, and whether the improvement in symptoms is worth the cost of the intervention.

- If there is marked symptom improvement throughout the
  trial, consider making this intervention a permanent part
  of your lifestyle.

CHAPTER 2 TO-DOS

- ☐ Ask your doctor to review all your labs and be certain you have a copy
  of them.

- ☐ Check with your health insurance company about coverage and copays for the
  various thyroid blood tests and about finding in-network healthcare providers.

- Talk to your insurance company about coverage for alternative healthcare practices that may interest you such as acupuncture, massage therapy, or chiropractic care.

- Set up a second appointment with your doctor if further questions arise after you have had time to think after your visit.

- Talk to your healthcare provider about additional labs that might be necessary, such as TSH, T4, T3, TPO antibody, and Tg tests.

- If you've had these labs, talk to your doctor about them to make sure you understand what they mean.

- If you suspect coexisting conditions, talk to your doctor about testing for these.

- Be honest about how you are feeling emotionally, as mental health issues can mimic Hashimoto's disease, and tell your doctor, nurse practitioner, or therapist. Your mind and body are connected (see chapter 4), so don't ignore your mental health.

- Practice saying no to others and assemble your Hashimoto's team, including support from family and friends.

DAILY CHECK-IN

Pausing to check in with your body is helpful in tracking your health.

- Scan your body and notice any physical sensations.

- Turn your attention inward and notice any thoughts or feelings that come up.

- Remember that changes to your diet, stress levels, or rest can affect how you're feeling right now.

- Do something nice for yourself to cultivate feelings of well-being.

3

EATING WELL WITH HASHIMOTO'S

No current scientific study-based evidence exists to support a Hashimoto's diet. However, many people living with Hashimoto's, including me, report feeling better when they eat a clean, anti-inflammatory diet. For conditions frequently coexisting with Hashimoto's, such as celiac disease or rheumatoid arthritis, dietary changes may be helpful. The plan outlined in this book has helped me, and many others, reduce and manage symptoms.

Your immune system needs adequate micronutrients (vitamins and minerals) and macronutrients (carbohydrates, fats, and proteins) to function properly. When you have autoimmune disease, you also need to eat foods that don't trigger inflammation, are low in contaminants, support healing, and provide nourishment.

Likewise, when you have autoimmune disease, it helps to eliminate foods that trigger immune responses, such as common allergens and foods to which you are sensitive. Having an immune response may cause flare-ups of symptoms and increase inflammation in sensitive individuals, particularly those with Hashimoto's.

This plan eliminates or minimizes most of the "Big 8" allergens (dairy, wheat, eggs, tree nuts, peanuts, shellfish, fish, and soy) as well as other inflammatory foods, including processed and genetically modified foods (GMOs), nightshades (certain plants), alcohol, and caffeine. For the most part, what you'll be doing is eating clean. If that sounds like a lot, don't worry. You'll still consume delicious and healthy foods, including animal proteins, fresh fruits and vegetables, fermented foods, and non-gluten whole grains.

Three Approaches to Clean

Clean means exactly what it sounds like: eating foods from nature in their purest form. There are three popular dietary approaches to clean feeding of the immune system:

- **The Mediterranean diet** is often recommended for people who seek a heart-healthy diet. Recipes for this diet contain complex carbohydrates, are low in sodium, and offer healthy fats.

- **The Paleo diet** uses recipes that are free of grain, sugar, dairy, processed ingredients, and industrial seed oils, and its focus is on whole foods found in nature. This diet can be a good choice for people with non-Hashimoto's autoimmune conditions, people who don't tolerate grains well, and people with diabetes.

- **The vegan diet** cuts out all animal products, which is attractive for people with a moral objection to the consumption of animals, or who just don't like the taste.

The recipes in this book contain an integration of all three approaches. Feel free to tailor your plan to your own specific preferences and circumstances.

GUIDELINES FOR CLEAN EATING

Keep these general guidelines in mind and you'll make a clean sweep in winning your food battles:

- Choose organic whenever possible, especially for foods that appear on the Dirty Dozen list (see Appendix B).
- Select organic, pastured animal proteins.
- Opt for wild-caught seafood.
- Choose nutrient-dense foods first.
- Read labels on packaged foods to avoid artificial and refined ingredients.

Dietary Recommendations for Hashimoto's

The following recommendations may help you achieve better thyroid health and an alleviation of symptoms:

- Eat an adequate amount of protein every day. The USDA recommends eating 0.36 gram of protein per pound of body weight on a daily basis.
- Minimize intake of goitrogens, which are foods that may have a negative impact on thyroid health. These include soy as well as raw cruciferous vegetables like Brussels sprouts, kale, broccoli, broccolini, turnips, collards, and cauliflower (cooked are okay).
- Exposure to mercury may decrease your body's production of thyroid hormones, according to a survey in *Environmental Health Perspectives*. Therefore, you may want to avoid foods that may contain high levels of mercury, particularly fish such as tuna or swordfish.
- Make nutrient-dense vegetables and fruit the basis of your diet. Eat a variety of plant foods across the spectrum of color to ensure you are well nourished and get all the vitamins and minerals you need.

- Because celiac disease—an autoimmune disease that occurs when ingesting gluten elicits an immune response that attacks the small intestine—and non-celiac gluten sensitivity are both conditions that occur frequently with thyroid disease, avoid gluten grains (wheat, rye, and barley, as well as oats manufactured in a facility that also processes gluten).
- Avoid dairy products because of high amounts of casein, a protein found in mammalian milk. Dairy allergies are largely associated with casein and often occur in conjunction with Hashimoto's.
- Avoid phytoestrogens in foods (soy, tempeh, sesame seeds). A 2011 study in the *Journal of Clinical Endocrinology & Metabolism* found an increase in the development of hypothyroidism in people who supplemented with soy.

Nutritional Considerations

A number of studies have shown that nutrient deficiencies can affect the body's use of thyroid hormones, the additional hormones the body produces, and thyroid medication. That's why ensuring you consume adequate amounts of nutrients every day is key to better health. The foods recommended as part of this plan contain adequate levels of vitamins and minerals important to synthesizing your thyroid hormones. Let's look at them individually.

Fiber

Eating a high-fiber diet can change how efficiently and quickly your body absorbs your thyroid medication. Increased dietary fiber is a great diet idea, and dosage adjustments are manageable. If you don't notice a significant change in symptoms and you are eating a high-fiber diet, talk to your doctor about managing your medication and diet.

Iron

Not having enough iron in your blood is just one potential form of anemia. Many kinds of anemia cause fatigue and weakness.

A study published in the *Biomedical Journal* (2015) noted that there is a high prevalence of iron deficiency in women with thyroid disease. To get the most from your thyroid hormones, it is important you maintain a healthy iron status, something that may be difficult for people with hypothyroidism.

If you are eating animal proteins, chances are you are getting adequate levels of iron in your diet. In the event you do require supplementation, do not take iron supplements within four hours of taking your thyroid medications, or else the iron supplement will not allow good thyroid absorption. Instead, consider taking your iron supplements in the evening, and your thyroid meds the following morning.

Copper

Copper helps your body produce thyroid-stimulating hormone (TSH). According to a 1999 article in the *British Medical Bulletin*, inadequate intake of copper can adversely affect thyroid function. A more recent study in the June 2014 issue of *Biological Trace Element Research* examined how the status of several minerals, including copper, affected thyroid function. Copper intake was associated with higher levels of thyroid hormones T3 and T4.

Foods high in copper include pumpkin and squash seeds, dark leafy greens, and asparagus.

Selenium

Your body needs the mineral selenium in trace amounts. An article in the February 2013 issue of *Clinical Endocrinology* looks at selenium status in autoimmune hypothyroidism (Hashimoto's), showing that selenium decreases antibodies that attack the thyroid, which may help minimize damage to the thyroid. Practitioner Chris Kresser, of the California Center for Functional Medicine, explains that selenium can also help your body use iodine efficiently while providing protection from exposure to too much iodine. This information is backed up by an earlier study in the October 2002 issue of the journal *Thyroid*.

How selenium interacts with iodine and impacts your thyroid is complex and an area of ongoing research. Aside from keeping some naturally selenium-rich foods in your diet, such as Brazil nuts or cremini mushrooms, it's best to include your doctor in any discussion of selenium supplementation, or before including additional selenium in your health plan. It's important you don't overdo it, because selenium can be toxic in high doses.

Vitamin B_{12}

More than 25 percent of people with hypothyroidism have vitamin B_{12} deficiency. It could be because the absorption of vitamin B_{12} is complicated. First, there is limited availability of B_{12} in non-meat foods. Vegans struggle to find natural sources of the vitamin, which is plentiful in animal proteins, including red meat, organ meats, poultry, eggs, and fish, although they can get B_{12} from nutritional yeast.

The second reason vitamin B_{12} is difficult to absorb is because it requires powerful hydrochloric acid in the stomach. Reduced gut acid can be a problem in those with malnourishment, previous stomach surgery, *H. pylori* bacteria, older age, certain acid blockers, and insulin resistance medication. The third possible complication to absorption is autoantibody production. In pernicious anemia, antibodies attack gut cells and block B_{12} absorption. Regular vitamin injections must be provided instead.

YOU Are a Priority

As a busy mom, volunteer, and professional writer, I understand how difficult it can be to prioritize—and even make some "me time." But I learned that for my best symptom management, I need to take time for myself each day. Making that happen can be tough, but it gets easier over time and with practice. To start, look for some creative ways to carve out small pockets of time, perhaps starting with just 30 minutes and building toward 60 to 90 minutes per day. Below are some ideas that have worked for me:

- If you can't take long breaks, schedule 10- to 15-minute blocks throughout the day, whenever you can get a little time for yourself.
- Set your alarm to wake you 15 minutes before everyone else, and allot meditation or relaxation time.
- Set up a babysitting cooperative, taking turns with one or two friends to provide each of you with an hour or two of respite.
- Make "no" part of your vocabulary. It's good to help out from time to time, but it's also okay to pass on PTA fundraisers, being team mom, hosting a jewelry party, or cooking for a major holiday.
- If you're driving kids to and fro, when you're alone in the car, practice mindfulness:
  - Eliminate distracting thoughts or emotions by keeping your attention on the present moment.
  - Notice the physical sights, sounds, smells, and textures around you.
  - Name what you are doing by using short words or phrases, like, "I'm driving slowly" or "Now I am braking."
  - Make a conscious effort to drive in as relaxed a manner as possible.

Vitamin D

Contrary to its name, technically, vitamin D isn't a vitamin—it's a steroid hormone produced by the body when it's exposed to sunshine. Over 90 percent of the vitamin D in the human body is produced by sunlight. Our bones need vitamin D, because without it, calcium can't do its job. A study in the *International Journal of Health Sciences* (2013) showed that people with hypothyroidism have significantly lower levels of vitamin D in their blood, and that the lower the levels, the more severe the symptoms of the hypothyroidism.

These days we don't absorb nearly enough sunlight to manufacture an adequate amount—and during winter, most of the country sees so little daylight that doing so seems impossible. Fortunately, you can boost your vitamin D levels by getting some unprotected sun exposure safely. The most common recommendation is 10 to 15 minutes on your arms and legs every day, or by taking a supplement. Talk to your doctor about your supplementation options.

It may be tempting to take supplements to support your diet. However, because Hashimoto's presents so differently in people, and because coexisting health conditions can affect your nutritional needs differently, you should work with a qualified nutrition practitioner before taking *any* supplements. They can run appropriate tests and help you work up an individualized plan for both foods and nutrients.

THE ELIMINATION DIET

Even people with the same condition may have different food triggers that cause symptoms. For example, I must avoid dairy and gluten, while my friend with Hashimoto's does just fine with both. It took a systematic process of assessing my diet for me to learn my food triggers, and you can do the same with an elimination diet. Learning your food triggers is an empowering way to manage your symptoms, because you can tailor the diet to your own unique needs—it isn't one-size-fits-all. Once you've identified your triggers, you'll be far less likely to experience unexpected bouts of symptoms, which is a wonderful thing.

How It Works

An elimination diet is pretty simple. First, you eliminate every possible trigger. With five or fewer ingredients, the recipes in this book, and the accompanying shopping lists, already do that for you. After four weeks, you can begin to add back foods one at a time and track your symptoms. To follow an elimination diet and determine your own triggers:

1. Track your symptoms for a couple of weeks before you begin the diet. (I find it's pretty easy to forget symptoms, or just forget how severe they were, once you start to feel better.) Keep a daily journal of how you feel or use the Symptom Tracker on page 76, and note any unusual flare-ups.

2. Follow the diet in this book for four weeks. Keep a daily journal of your symptoms. By the end of four weeks, you should notice they have lessened significantly.

3. After four weeks, add one food back into your diet. For instance, try adding milk. Drink milk (or use another dairy product) and note your symptoms. If you remain symptom-free after 24 hours, try ingesting it again daily for one week and track your symptoms. If the symptoms recur, you can assume that this food is a trigger. If they don't, then the food is likely not a trigger.

4. Don't introduce more than one food category (see pages 60 to 69) per week. Slow reintroduction of foods will avoid shocking your system and will allow you to ascertain which foods are causing your issues.

FOODS TO AVOID OR LIMIT

During the first phase of the elimination diet, you will be avoiding or limiting many foods listed in this section.

Alcohol

According to the National Institute on Alcohol Abuse and Alcoholism, alcohol consumption increases inflammation and weakens the immune system. Likewise, it can cause sleep disturbances, has profound effects on the brain, and can cause damage to other organs. Because it has so many potential deleterious effects, it is important that, while on the elimination diet, you avoid alcohol in all its forms, including wine, beer, hard liquor, and mixed drinks. Additionally, because many of your symptoms may include mental-emotional ones, it is critical to not use any mind-altering substances that may heighten already existing bad feelings, or induce them.

Corn

It's shocking how much corn, or corn-derived products, people eat in a standard Western diet. Corn is ubiquitous. Aside from the golden morsels we coat with butter and eat off cobs, corn products are used in many baked goods, sodas, condiments, juices, animal feed, and an entire array of refined and processed foods. It is a popular filler in many animal and synthetic products and is likely to be genetically modified (GMO). Highly inflammatory and a common allergen, corn also raises blood sugar rapidly, which can contribute to inflammation.

Foods to Avoid

- Artificial coloring
- Artificial sweeteners
- Baked goods
- Candy
- Corn: canned, frozen, on the cob
- Corn chips
- Corn-fed animals
- Cornstarch
- Corn syrup
- Juice, sweetened
- Masa
- Popcorn
- Soda
- Tamales
- Tortillas

Dairy

Dairy products are a common allergen. People may be sensitive to dairy in more than one way. For example, some people are sensitive to a sugar in the milk called lactose. Lactose intolerance can cause gastric distress. The other common sensitivity to dairy is an allergy to casein, which is a protein in milk. I am allergic to casein and experience inflammation and respiratory distress when I ingest milk, but I am not sensitive to lactose. Some people are unlucky enough to be sensitive to both. But no matter how you're affected, it's best to avoid dairy until you are certain you don't have issues.

Foods to Avoid

- Baked goods
- Butter
- Buttermilk
- Candy
- Caramels
- Cheese
- Cocoa
- Cream (half-and-half and heavy cream)
- Custard
- Ice cream
- Margarine
- Milk
- Milk chocolate
- Nougat
- Pudding
- Salad dressings (ranch, blue cheese, and others containing dairy—check the label)
- Whey
- Whipped cream
- Whipped topping
- White sauces
- Yogurt

Feedlot Animal Products

Factory-farmed animals tend to harbor more toxins and less nutrition than pasture-raised animals. According to a review in *Nutrition Journal,* pasture-raised animals are nutritionally superior in a number of ways, including:

- higher in omega-3 fatty acids
- higher concentration of antioxidants
- raised without hormones or antibiotics
- meat lower in fat and calories

In addition, crowded and unsanitary conditions in feedlots may result in higher levels of foodborne bacteria in the resulting meat, according to many studies, including one published in the *Canadian Veterinary Journal* (2009).

Select pasture-raised (also called pastured, grass-fed, or free-range) animal proteins, including eggs, poultry, beef, lamb, and pork.

Keep an Eye Out

Unless otherwise noted on the package, some products are commonly made from feedlot animals. These include:

- conventionally raised livestock
- conventionally raised poultry
- hot dogs
- processed meats such as cold cuts, which may also contain sugar, salt, and preservatives
- sausage, bacon, and other meats high in sulfites

Peanuts

Peanuts are a common allergen that can cause a severe reaction in some people. However, even if you don't experience a severe reaction, you may be sensitive to peanuts and have an inflammatory reaction.

Foods to Avoid

- Baked goods containing peanuts or peanut butter
- Candies
- Mixed nuts
- Peanut butter
- Peanuts
- Trail mix

Processed Foods

Processed foods are often high in sugar, salt, refined grains, refined oils, artificial colors and flavors, and chemical preservatives. In other words, many processed foods contain ingredients that aren't really food at all. Processed foods typically come in bags, boxes, cartons, and cans, and you may not be able to pronounce some of the ingredients listed on their labels. These include baked goods, chips, soups and stews, frozen meals, crackers, candy, condiments, fast food, and hundreds of other foods that often form the basis of the standard Western diet.

Due to the nature of their ingredients, processed foods can trigger inflammation and cause rapid rises in blood sugar. Depending on the ingredients, processed foods may contribute to the development of other types of diseases. Furthermore, processed foods tend to be high in calories but relatively low in nutrients, making them a poor choice for good health.

Soy

Soy is a phytoestrogen and a goitrogen, both of which can negatively impact thyroid health. While it's not proof, I can relate a personal story: Back when I was still struggling to figure out what was wrong with my health, I tried a number of diets. For about two years, I was a vegan and consumed a lot of tofu. It was during that period that I gained the most weight and struggled with a severe worsening of my thyroid symptoms.

Foods to Avoid

- Bean sprouts
- Edamame
- Hydrolyzed plant protein
- Hydrolyzed soy protein
- Soybean oil
- Soymilk
- Tempeh
- Tofu

Sugar and Chemical Artificial Sweeteners

Studies have linked sugar consumption to everything from diabetes and obesity to cancer and heart disease. It may also increase inflammation, and it triggers a rapid rise of blood glucose. Likewise, sugar is non-nutritive—that is, it contains calories without any vitamins or minerals to nourish your body. Unfortunately, in the Western world we have developed a mighty craving for sweetness and sugar, and it is pervasive in processed foods. Read the label on most processed foods, and you'll find some form of sugar somewhere in the ingredient list, including in savory foods like soups and stews where you wouldn't think there'd be any.

Food manufacturers' answer to sugar is artificial sweeteners: highly sweet chemical substances that don't contain calories in an average-size serving. This includes aspartame (NutraSweet), sucralose (Splenda), cyclamate (Sugar Twin), acesulfame K (acesulfame potassium), and saccharine. These are all chemicals not natural for human consumption, and they can trigger inflammation. For the recipes in this book, a natural sweetener extracted from stevia will be used.

Wheat and Gluten Grains

Many people with Hashimoto's are sensitive to wheat and gluten grains. Some people may have celiac disease, in which ingestion of gluten can cause severe damage to the intestines, leading to malabsorption of nutrients, gastric distress, and inflammation. People may also have non-celiac gluten sensitivity, which can cause reactions like gastrointestinal distress and inflammation. Likewise, wheat is inflammatory for many people, and a common allergen.

Foods to Avoid

- Baked goods
- Barley
- Breakfast cereals
- Chips
- Crackers
- Durum
- Flour
- Gravy
- Malt
- Oats (unless certified as gluten-free)
- Pasta
- Prepared mustard (if it contains wheat— check the label)
- Pretzels
- Processed foods
- Rye

- Salad dressing and marinades (check the label for artificial and gluten ingredients)
- Seitan
- Semolina
- Soy sauce (unless certified as gluten-free)
- Spelt
- Surimi (imitation crab meat)
- Wheat
- Wheat germ

FOODS TO AVOID NOW BUT MAY BE REINTRODUCED LATER

Eating of foods in this section will be limited for the elimination diet, but as you move forward after your four weeks, you can try them. Not everyone is reactive to these foods, although some people will be. In the best interests of your health, reintroduce them slowly and see how you fare.

Citrus Fruits

Citrus fruits are high in sugar, which can be an issue when you are trying to fight inflammation. While some recipes may call for a small amount of freshly squeezed lemon or lime juice, or zest from peels, a whole piece of citrus or its juice is too high in sugar for the purposes of this plan.

Citrus to Avoid for Now

- Grapefruit and grapefruit juice
- Kumquats
- Oranges and orange juice
- Pomelo
- Satsuma
- Tangelo
- Tangerines and tangerine juice
- Ugli fruit
- Yuzu

Fish and Shellfish

Freshwater and saltwater fish are a common food allergen, with about 0.4 percent of the US population reporting an allergy to fish, according to the *Journal of Allergy and Clinical Immunology*. Shellfish allergies are even more common, with a prevalence of about 2 percent.

Just because you are allergic to fish does not mean you are allergic to shellfish, or vice versa, but about 0.2 percent of the population in the United States is allergic to both. Because they are such a common allergen, you should avoid both fish and shellfish. When you reintroduce them, consider them separate categories. As discussed previously, you should also avoid fish that are at high risk of mercury contamination (see page 54).

Fish to Avoid for Now

- Anchovies
- Arctic char
- Bass
- Cod (including cod liver oil)
- Haddock
- Halibut
- Herring
- John Dory
- Mackerel
- Mahi mahi
- Orange roughy
- Salmon
- Sardines
- Steelhead trout
- Swordfish
- Trout
- Tuna

Shellfish to Avoid for Now

- Abalone
- Clams
- Crab
- Crawfish
- Krill (including krill oil)
- Langostino
- Mussels
- Octopus
- Scallops
- Shrimp/prawns
- Squid/calamari

Nightshades

Some people with autoimmune disease react to a category of plant foods called nightshades, a botanical designation for a large family of flowering plants that contain chemicals called saponins, lectins, and capsaicin. These chemicals protect the plants against predators but may act as a mild irritant when we eat them, leading to inflammation and other issues, particularly in people with autoimmune disease. Therefore, eliminating nightshades to start is essential, but you may be able to reintroduce them. I don't have a problem with nightshades, and was able to reintroduce them successfully after my elimination diet, which made me very happy because I adore hot chile peppers and tomatoes.

Nightshades to Avoid for Now

- Bell peppers
- Cayenne
- Chile peppers
- Chili powder
- Eggplant
- Goji berries
- Gooseberries
- Paprika
- Potatoes (except sweet potatoes)
- Sriracha hot sauce
- Tomatillos
- Tomatoes

Pulses/Legumes

Pulses and legumes may cause an inflammation reaction in some people, so it's best to limit them on the elimination diet.

Pulses/Legumes to Avoid for Now

- Chickpeas
- Fava beans
- Kidney beans
- Lentils
- Lima beans
- Navy beans
- Peas

Tree Nuts

Tree nuts are one of the Big 8 allergens (the most commonly occurring food allergies), affecting between 25 and 40 percent of the population, according to the American College of Allergy, Asthma, and Immunology. Allergies can be mild and include gastrointestinal or respiratory symptoms, or they can be quite severe, causing anaphylaxis.

Tree Nuts to Avoid for Now

- Almonds
- Brazil nuts
- Cashews
- Chestnuts
- Hazelnuts (filberts)
- Macadamia nuts
- Pecans
- Pine nuts
- Pistachios
- Walnuts

FOODS TO ENJOY

After reading the list of foods to eliminate, you may be feeling a bit worried, which is perfectly natural. After all, just the words "elimination diet" bring to mind deprivation. I have good news, however. Even though you will be eliminating certain foods—some temporarily and some permanently—there are plenty of delicious and healthy foods you can eat that will provide you with a tasty, richly varied diet of easy-to-prepare foods. Consider this an opportunity to try wonderful new flavor combinations (I'm sure some will become new favorites). The foods you can eat are rich in nutrients and loaded with flavor, and will help nourish and sustain your body as you begin your journey to good health.

Fruits and Vegetables

One of the great things about our food system in the Western world is that we have a variety of fruits and vegetables available year-round. While I always recommend that for the peak of flavor and nutrition you try to incorporate local and seasonal fruits and

whenever you can (check out local farmers' markets
nity-supported agriculture programs), even in the
inter you can find plenty of delicious produce at your
ery store.

Fruits to Enjoy

Limit fruits to one or two servings per day to minimize
sugar intake.

- Apples
- Apricots
- Avocado
- Bananas
- Berries
- Cherries
- Coconut
- Figs
- Grapes
- Kiwis
- Mango
- Melons
- Nectarines
- Papaya
- Peaches
- Pears
- Pineapple
- Plums
- Pluots (a cross between a plum and an apricot)
- Pomegranate

Vegetables and Tubers to Enjoy

Whether you eat them raw or cooked, vegetables and tubers are
loaded with nutrients, vitamins, minerals, and antioxidants. Try to
incorporate several servings of vegetables into your daily routine.

- Asparagus
- Beets
- Carrots
- Celery
- Cucumbers
- Fennel
- Green beans
- Jicama
- Leafy greens such as spinach and lettuce
- Mushrooms
- Onions
- Scallions
- Shallots

- Summer squash (zucchini, pattypan squash, yellow squash, etc.)
- Sweet potatoes/yams
- Turnips/rutabagas (cooked)
- Winter squash (acorn squash, spaghetti squash, butternut squash, etc.)

Animal Proteins

Animal foods provide an excellent source of protein, which is essential for muscle building and repair. Try to select naturally raised, pastured animal proteins.

Animal Proteins to Enjoy

- Beef
- Eggs
- Game meats
- Lamb
- Organ meats
- Pork
- Poultry (chicken, duck, turkey)

Grains

While this diet eliminates a lot of grains, you can still enjoy some. If you choose to include grains, limit intake to about ½ cup per day.

Grains to Enjoy

- Oats (certified gluten-free)
- Quinoa
- Rice

Herbs and Spices

Herbs and spices make everything delicious. Many, such as ginger and turmeric, also have wonderful healing and anti-inflammatory properties that support good health and well-being.

Herbs and Spices to Enjoy

- Allspice
- Basil
- Black pepper
- Caraway

- Cardamom
- Cilantro
- Cinnamon
- Citrus zest
- Cloves
- Coriander
- Cumin
- Curry
- Dill
- Fennel seed
- Garlic
- Ginger
- Mustard powder
- Nutmeg
- Oregano
- Parsley
- Rosemary
- Saffron
- Sage
- Sea salt
- Tarragon
- Thyme
- Turmeric

Fats and Oils

Fats and oils are an important part of the diet. They play critical roles in the body, including providing energy and allowing you to absorb certain nutrients. The type of fatty acid you consume also affects inflammation: omega-3 fatty acids are anti-inflammatory, while omega-6 fatty acids cause inflammation. While you need both types of fatty acids for optimal health (as inflammation is an important and necessary function of the immune system), the standard Western diet is very high in omega-6 fatty acids and low in omega-3 fatty acids. This imbalance leads to chronic inflammation, which plays a significant role in autoimmune diseases, including Hashimoto's thyroiditis.

One of the reasons the omega-3 to omega-6 ratio is so unbalanced in the standard Western diet is the heavy use of industrial seed oils, which tend to be very high in omega-6 fatty acids. Industrial seed oils include canola oil, sunflower oil, safflower oil, refined sesame oil, cotton oil, and similar refined oils. To help balance fatty acid profiles, this plan uses more natural oils and fats, such as expeller-pressed (not refined) oils as well as fats from animal sources, which provide nourishment and minimize inflammation.

Fats and Oils to Enjoy

- Avocado oil (expeller-pressed)
- Coconut oil
- Duck fat
- Extra-virgin olive oil
- Lard from pastured animals
- Schmaltz (chicken fat)
- Sesame oil (expeller-pressed)
- Tallow from pastured animals
- Flaxseed oil (as a supplement)

Other Foods

Other foods that you can enjoy—and that are included in the recipes in this book—include:

- Apple juice (unsweetened)
- Applesauce (unsweetened)
- Broth (chicken, beef, vegetable)
- Coconut milk
- Coconut yogurt (plain)
- Dijon mustard (wheat-free)
- Fermented foods (such as pickles, sauerkraut, gluten-free soy sauce, and fish sauce)
- Seeds (such as chia, flaxseed, pumpkin seeds, and sunflower seeds)
- Sunflower butter

This list doesn't contain all the foods you can eat, but it gives you a good idea of the categories and some of the foods that fall into them. Every person is different with individual tolerances, so it's important to check in with your symptoms and track any foods that may trigger reactions. This is particularly true when you begin reintroducing foods to your diet, but you should also listen to your body while you are on the elimination diet, watching to ensure that you don't have any uncommon sensitivities.

FOOD REINTRODUCTION AND SYMPTOM TRACKER

After four weeks on the meal plan, and assuming you are seeing an improvement in your symptoms, you can start carefully reintroducing foods into your diet to see what works for you. Reintroduce foods in any order you prefer, but add only one food at a time, and allow at least a week before moving on to the next. During that week, carefully track any and all symptoms you experience. Foods to reintroduce include:

- Citrus
- Fish
- Nightshades
- Pulses/legumes
- Shellfish
- Tree nuts

Foods you need to continue to avoid include:

- Alcohol
- Caffeine
- Corn
- Dairy
- Feedlot animal products
- Gluten grains/wheat
- Peanuts
- Processed foods
- Soy

Although avoidance is best, some people do choose to reintroduce the above foods into their diet. If you do so, consume them only in extremely limited amounts. For example, I eat cleanly more than 95 percent of the time. Perhaps once a month, or less frequently, I may have a small serving of one of the foods I avoid, such as alcohol. I never have wheat or gluten due to my celiac disease, but occasionally a bit of dairy may slip in. Because I eat so cleanly the rest of the time, I suffer only mild symptoms from eating these foods. Even so, I give myself plenty of recovery time by eating the most nourishing foods I can find in the days and weeks that follow.

For some people, the plan may take longer than four weeks. If you aren't noticing any change in symptoms at the end of that time, continue the elimination diet for another two to four weeks.

When symptoms resolve, then you can begin to reintroduce foods. Bodies heal in their own time, and some people may need more time than others. It took me about three months on the elimination diet before I felt well enough to begin reintroducing foods, but I had 25 years of damage from illness to repair. Be patient and give your body the time it needs to heal. Listen to what your body has to tell you.

Step-by-Step Food Challenges

Here's how to reintroduce food back into your diet:

1. Choose one category of food, such as tree nuts. Pick one tree nut, such as almond.

2. Before you eat any almonds, record any symptoms you have, noting the severity.

3. Eat a few almonds. Note how you feel throughout the day, but don't eat any more.

4. Note how you feel the next day. If you still feel well, eat a few more almonds or try a tablespoon of almond butter.

5. For one week, track your symptoms as you continue to eat a small amount of almonds each day. If your symptoms return at any time, stop eating the almonds and return to your elimination diet until your symptoms disappear. Then reintroduce another category of foods.

6. After one week, if you don't have symptoms, then you may assume you are not sensitive to almonds.

7. Next (only if you had no symptoms), try another tree nut, such as walnut or pecan, following the above steps. If you make it through the week without symptoms, it is safe to assume you are not allergic to tree nuts, and you can add the entire category back into your dietary rotation.

8. Repeat the process for each food category, trying two or three foods before assuming that you aren't sensitive to that category. For example, if you are reintroducing nightshades, try tomatoes, then potatoes, and then chile peppers, which will take

Tracking Your Symptoms

Symptom Tracker

Time Period	Symptoms (bloating, diarrhea, cramps, etc.)	Severity of Symptoms (on a scale of 1 to 10)
Baseline		
End of Week 1		
End of Week 2		
End of Week 3		
End of Week 4		

Have your symptoms alleviated? If not, continue the diet for another two to four weeks. If you still don't see progress, consult your doctor, dietician, or other medical professional for additional advice.

Food Challenges Tracker

Food Category	Food Item & Serving Size	Date & Time Consumed	Symptoms	Conclusion
Tree Nuts	*5 almonds*	*Sun. @ noon*	*Hives, bloating*	*Must avoid* ✗
Night-shades	*2 cherry tomatoes*	*Fri. @ 7 p.m.*	*No problems!*	*Okay to eat* ✓

about three weeks. If you show any sensitivity to one item from a category, stop trying to reintroduce foods from that category, assume you are sensitive to it, and eliminate it permanently. Once symptoms disappear, move on to the next category.

What If It Doesn't Work?

In some cases, the elimination diet may not provide relief from your symptoms, even after several months. This may occur for a number of reasons:

- You have coexisting conditions that are causing symptoms, such as other autoimmune conditions, iron deficiency anemia, or pernicious anemia.
- Your body may just be slow in healing. If this is the case, considerable time may pass before you notice subtle changes in symptoms.
- You may have some unusual food sensitivity or allergy that is stalling your progress.
- Eggs are a common allergen that this diet doesn't exclude. You may be allergic to them and may wish to try and eliminate them as well.
- You may be taking medications or using substances that are stalling your progress. For example, if you're a smoker, note that tobacco is a nightshade.
- During food prep, you may be cross-contaminating yourself with allergens such as gluten or nuts.
- Your Hashimoto's diagnosis may not be correct.

If All Else Fails

If you don't see some improvement after several weeks on the diet, try the following:

- First, double-check to make sure that you haven't cross-contaminated yourself from gluten or other allergen residue. Visit a celiac disease website, such as celiac.com, to learn how to set up your kitchen to avoid cross-contamination.

- If cross-contamination isn't the issue, it may be time to visit your doctor again. Have your iron levels checked and ask that an allergy scratch test be performed.

- You may also wish to connect with a good source of thyroid information, such as stopthethyroidmadness.com, where you can hear from other people with Hashimoto's and learn about the things that have helped them minimize symptoms and feel better. There are also a number of Hashimoto's support groups available that are a good source of information.

- Self-advocacy is extremely important, so informing yourself as much as possible can be helpful in getting to the bottom of your unique health situation. I finally got a proper diagnosis because I learned everything I could and advocated for myself. This is something you too can do.

CHAPTER 3 TO-DOS

☐ Make a copy of the Symptom Tracker (see page 76) and start tracking symptoms right away.

☐ Make a copy of the "Foods to Enjoy" chart (see Appendix A) and put it where you can study it frequently.

☐ Set up your kitchen for success, getting rid of foods you won't be eating any longer.

☐ Begin stocking your kitchen with healthy foods.

☐ Set a start date for your four-week elimination diet plan.

☐ If you share the kitchen with gluten or allergen eaters, set up a gluten- and allergen-free zone. Designate one or two cupboards for gluten- or allergen-containing foods, as well as other foods that aren't on your plan. Designate counter space where others prepare their gluten- or allergen-containing foods, and use all other counter space for your food prep, to avoid cross-contamination.

☐ Learn protocols to avoid cross-contamination from allergens.

DAILY CHECK-IN

Pausing to check in with your body is helpful in tracking your health.

- ☐ Scan your body and notice any physical sensations.
- ☐ Turn your attention inward and notice any thoughts or feelings that come up.
- ☐ Remember that changes to your diet, stress levels, or rest can affect how you're feeling right now.
- ☐ Do something nice for yourself to cultivate feelings of well-being.

4

LIVING WELL WITH HASHIMOTO'S

It used to be considered alternative or new-agey to suggest that treating physical illness required equal attention and care to the mind; that somehow what the body feels, so does the mind, and what the mind experiences manifests in the body. Known as the mind-body connection, scores of people from the most credentialed medical experts at top medical centers to the pedestrian patient now are convinced of the existence of such a connection. The connection suggests that when you are ill, doing your due diligence to tend to your physical body and addressing the components that cause your symptoms is not enough. The mind is very much tied into how you feel physically, and vice versa. Think about the last time you felt at your lowest. Didn't you also feel depressed, hopeless, anxious? And how about the last time you felt overly stressed or unusually peaceful? Did you take note of your physical symptoms that day? The mind and the body are interconnected and interdependent. No doubt about it. Developing habits that bridge the gap between your mind and body is critical in your Hashimoto's journey, so let's get started.

We exist in a high-stress world, living life at top speed. The pressures of job, family, and society can seem overwhelming, particularly when you're also dealing with a chronic illness, which is a stress all by itself.

Stress isn't necessarily a bad thing. In fact, it's a natural part of the human existence. According to the American Psychological Association, stress is an important part of the human "fight or flight" response, which was once necessary when early humans were prey to large and dangerous predators. When faced with the stress of becoming someone's dinner, early humans were flooded with stress hormones that allowed them to either flee or fight for their lives so they didn't wind up a tasty snack.

Unfortunately, even though humans seldom encounter the risk of becoming prey any longer, we still have a pretty powerful stress response. And in this day and age of stressful living, our stress may be chronic, so we have a constant flurry of stress hormones flowing through our bodies. Since stress hormones (like adrena-line) are designed to come quickly and go quickly, our modern-day stress preserves them steadily in our systems, causing unintended and negative effects on our health.

Psychology Today notes that chronic stress is very hard on the body, exacerbating existing conditions, causing headaches and pain, contributing to disease, increasing the risk of cardiac events, and impeding recovery from illness and injury.

The effects of chronic stress on the body are so catastrophic, in fact, that reducing stress is probably as important as changing your diet and taking your medication.

While my life certainly isn't stress-free, it's a lot better than it used to be. In my younger years, I was a stress monster. I worried nearly constantly and was on the go all the time, no matter how ill I felt. I was also a world-class procrastinator and a bit of a drama queen. With these behaviors, I kept myself in a constant state of stress. However, I soon learned and acknowledged how negatively stress affected my health, and began to change. Compared to that much younger version of me, I'm practically Zen these days, and it has made a huge impact on how I feel emotionally, physically, and spiritually. Along with helping my physical symptoms, it's also made my life more fulfilling in every single way: It's improved my relationships, helped me sleep better, made my work far more enjoyable, and enabled me to slow down and appreciate the beauty of the life I live.

Managing your stress can do similar things for you. It can help your health, your relationships, your job, and your appreciation of life. What could be better?

Strategies for Reducing Overall Stress

The strategies I implemented helped me transform from a stress monster to a Zen creature. You, too, can achieve peacefulness.

- **Define and protect your boundaries.** We've already talked a lot about the power of no, and when you're enforcing your boundaries, "no" becomes an important word. In order to be able to say no, however, you must first decide the things you want to say no to. These are your boundaries, and they arise from your values and your priorities. In a journal or on a piece of paper, take the time to determine exactly where your boundaries lie, and then begin gently enforcing them.

- **Know your physical and mental limits.** When you are dealing with chronic illness, you often have a limited amount of physical and mental resources. It's natural to try and override these and do too much, something I understand perfectly. However, when we try to exceed these limitations, we exact a price from our bodies and minds in terms of stress, increased symptoms, exhaustion, and similar issues. Therefore, it is important that you respect yourself enough not to push beyond these limitations in order to truly care for yourself.

- **Step away from negativity.** Sometimes, there are people in your life who take far more than they give, and boy, can they bring the drama! For your own health, whenever possible, step gently away from these people.

- *Find a calming activity you enjoy.* It can be a 15-minute walk, closing your eyes and breathing deeply, meditating, or any other calming activity, but taking a mental break is critical to living well with chronic stress and illness. I have several activities I enjoy: I make jewelry, write poetry, meditate, play the piano, read, and many others. Make time to engage in activities that you enjoy, even if it's for just a few moments a day.

- *Focus on the now.* I'm a big fan of remaining present-time focused, worrying as little as possible about the past or the future. Instead, pay attention to this very moment, noting all your senses and your feelings as you go through the day. Removing attention from the past and future is grounding and makes the now more vibrant and interesting.

As you work your way through the four-week plan, you'll receive specific suggestions for stress management that you can incorporate into your lifestyle.

THE PRACTICE OF SELF-COMPASSION

I consider self-compassion the key to a successful four-week plan and Hashimoto's lifestyle. It's the reason I started this book with a self-compassion exercise: Without being kind to yourself, you can't cross the threshold of inner wisdom and begin to heal. In the beginning of the book, we needed to learn how self-compassion moves us away from victimhood or self-blame and into a frame of mind of power and deserving better treatment; here we hone our self-compassion skills for the sake of our spirits, and because now we know how a positive mind can lead to a powerful body. That's what we want, after all, right?

Self-compassion, once you think about it, makes logical sense. Imagine a loved one comes to you with a serious issue. It is likely you respond with compassion and caring, offering empathy and kindness. You are there for your friend as a reliable presence to help her through her difficult time. You check in with her and send unsolicited text messages, just letting her know you are thinking

Mindfulness and Eating Meditation

Mindfulness helps you manage stress. It's a form of living meditation that focuses you on the present moment. Practicing mindfulness during eating can help you stick to your diet.

- Enjoy your meal free of distractions. Turn off the television and plan to just eat. Play some soft music, if you like.
- Notice the food on your plate. Observe the colors and shapes of the food.
- Express gratitude. Give thanks for the food that will nourish and support your body.
- Notice the aroma of the food, breathing deeply.
- Take a small forkful, allowing it to sit on your tongue as you notice the flavors and textures. Chew thoroughly, paying attention to how the flavors and textures change.
- Swallow and feel the food traveling down your throat. Imagine it moving throughout your body, providing nourishment and healing to every cell.
- Continue taking small bites and eating slowly, until you have finished your meal. Listen to your body's signals and stop eating if you feel full before your plate is empty.

Eating this way helps you slow down, relax, and focus on your physical, mental, and emotional well-being. Even if you feel that the meditation didn't "work," continue the practice. It offers an opportunity to slow down, lighten up, and cope with the stressors of life.

of her. You ask her over for tea and offer to pick up her kids from school, so she can have some alone time. Now think about a time when you were experiencing some difficulty. How did you treat yourself? Were you as kind and attentive to yourself as you were to your friend, or did you let your inner critic run free, placing blame and guilt on yourself and being generally unkind?

We all have an inner critic. I've even named mine Lillith. My inner critic is super mean and judgmental, telling me all sorts of things are my fault, criticizing me at the slightest mistake, and jeering at my reflection in the mirror on bad hair days. I used to pay a lot of attention to the things she said to me, and it always left me feeling awful and slightly nauseous.

Most people have a "Lillith," and the thoughts this inner judge shares are not usually kind or compassionate. In fact, the inner critic can be downright hostile, filling your mind full of your faults and shortcomings.

Many people think the inner critic exists to motivate them into action and help them be better people, but this is a fallacy. After all, how motivated would you feel if some stranger (or even worse, someone you care about) started yammering about all that is wrong with you? Such encounters are demoralizing, shaming, and discouraging, not supportive or encouraging. Yet this is what we do to ourselves on a regular basis as we listen to our inner critic.

Think of it this way: Would you talk to a loved one the way your inner critic talks to you? Chances are, unless you're a really mean person (and I doubt you are), you wouldn't! You would make every attempt to communicate with kindness and recognize your common humanity with the other person. And that's exactly how you should treat yourself.

This is the basis for the act of self-compassion. It's a way to talk and treat yourself with kindness, care, and compassion, and it is an important way of supporting yourself. You cannot get better, get focused, get well, without learning to kick your inner critic's butt and lock her out of your mind for good.

In her book, *Self-Compassion: The Proven Power of Being Kind to Yourself,* Kristin Neff, PhD, describes three essential components of self-compassion:

- **Self-kindness:** Treat yourself kindly, as you would treat someone else. This involves recognizing your own imperfections and failings and giving yourself a break by being gentle with yourself.

- **Common humanity:** Realize that you are human and recognize that you share suffering and human failings with all of humanity.

- **Mindfulness:** Allow yourself to experience your emotions without judging them or suppressing them. Instead, pay attention and allow yourself to experience emotions without commentary or judgment. By allowing yourself to experience your emotions fully without judgment, they pass through you and resolve.

This is how you treat others when you are being compassionate, and it is also how you should treat yourself. Consider how it would feel to silence your inner critic and simply allow yourself to feel how you feel without self-judgment.

The work of the author Byron Katie played a big role in helping me live more compassionately, both with myself and with others. Katie offers a simple process she calls "The Work," and when I started doing it several years ago, my inner critic fell silent. While you can read about Katie's work in her books or on her website, TheWork.com, doing the work, which is a process she calls inquiry, is quite simple and involves four simple questions that you ask whenever you find yourself judging yourself or another. Consider the judgment and ask yourself the following questions:

1. Is that true?
2. How can you possibly know that is true?
3. How do you react when you believe that thought?
4. Who would you be without that thought?

Soothing My Inner Critic

Our inner critic can be harsh and difficult to ignore, and when we get down on ourselves, the suffering can sometimes feel unbearable. So we may be surprised to know that our inner critic is a part of us, and it often acts the way it does because it cares and wants us to be safe. It is fearful for us, and so in its warped way, it thinks it is protecting us. It just doesn't know how to help in a constructive way.

So how do we quiet it? One way is to give the inner critic (that part of us that's afraid) compassion. To do this, try the following exercise in self-compassion, which has been adapted from the work of Kristin Neff and her book, *Self-Compassion*.

1. First, think of a common thing your inner critic says to you. Start with something small, one that involves an action that you have some control over. What kinds of words or tone does your inner critic use? *I am such an idiot for eating that snack. I have no willpower—what's WRONG with me? Why can't I do anything right? My inner critic uses a harsh, mean, judgmental tone.*

2. Now, describe how you feel when your inner critic talks to you this way. *I feel sad, despairing, disappointed in myself, guilty, hopeless.*

3. Picture your inner critic as the child version of you, sitting in your lap. Instead of trying to silence it, try to think about why it is saying these things. What is it afraid of, and what does it want or need? *My inner critic is scared that if I eat too much, I'll gain weight and feel worse about myself. My inner critic wants me to be healthy and happy with myself.*

4. Finish by offering your inner critic some compassion. What would you say to soothe this child sitting on your lap? *I am so sorry you are going through this. You must be so worried, and I know you're just trying to help. Thank you for caring about me and trying to help me be healthy. I hear what you're saying, and I'll try to do better next time.*

Now that you've gone through this once, how do you feel? You may be surprised to see that your inner critic wants the same things you do. It just hasn't learned the right ways of getting you there. The next time your inner critic hurts you, consider giving it (and therefore yourself) some self-compassion. You may be surprised by the results.

These four simple questions have made a profound difference in my life and how I perceive and interact with myself and others. This thoughtfulness with which I have learned to treat myself has allowed me to live a more present-time focused, loving, compassionate, caring, and stress-free life, and it can do the same for you. I strongly urge you to check out the work of both Kristin Neff and Byron Katie to help you learn to treat yourself more compassionately.

IMPROVING YOUR SLEEP HYGIENE

I have always been someone who needs a lot of sleep, and since my Hashimoto's kicked in, I've needed even more. I feel my best with at least eight solid hours of sleep per night.

Not everyone needs to sleep as much as I do, but most Americans need far more sleep than they are getting. Americans are chronically sleep deprived. According to the Better Sleep Council, adults need a solid eight hours of sleep per night, but a 2013 Gallup poll showed that the average American sleeps only about 6.8 hours, with more than 40 percent of Americans getting less than the recommended amount.

According to the Division of Sleep Medicine at the Harvard Medical School, health effects of chronic sleep deprivation can be brutal, and include decreased life expectancy, diseases, and circumstances putting you at risk for disease, including:

- Obesity
- Diabetes
- High blood pressure
- Heart disease
- Impaired immunity
- Mood disorders
- Overuse of alcohol

As someone with a chronic illness, getting adequate sleep (seven to nine hours) is especially important, because you need your body to be firing on all cylinders in order to stay as healthy as possible.

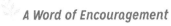 *A Word of Encouragement*

Chronic illness doesn't mean a life sentence of chronically feeling badly. By creating a series of personalized lifestyle and dietary modifications and listening to your body, you can improve your symptoms and your life. You may find this has been an unexpected opportunity to get acquainted with yourself in ways you wouldn't have otherwise. It's all about shifting your perspective. You can do it!

Strategies for Better Sleep Hygiene

In order to promote better and longer sleep, good sleep hygiene is essential. The Centers for Disease Control and Prevention (CDC) recommends several positive sleep habits that can promote better sleep:

- *Set the environment right for sleep.* Sleep in a dark room away from noise and light pollution. Make sure your bed and pillow are comfortable and keep the room at a comfortable temperature to avoid your body from becoming too hot or cold while asleep, causing you to wake. Remove distractions that might wake you, such as smartphones, pets, bright alarm clocks, or allergens, like flowers. Consider a white noise machine if you live in a noisy area or if your sleep partner is a snorer.

- *Go to bed every night at the same time and get up each morning at the same time.* Yes, this includes weekends. This regularity helps your body adapt to sleeping and trains it to expect to go to sleep and wake the same time every day, making the transition from sleeping to waking much easier. For me it's also had an added benefit: I don't need an alarm to wake up. My body (and my dogs) just knows when to do it.

- *Don't eat or drink right before bed.* The process of trying to digest food can disrupt sleep, as can issues related to eating so close to bed, such as heartburn or gas. And, of course, drinking before bed can result in a 3 a.m. bathroom run. Not good for restfulness.

- *Avoid alcohol and caffeine before bed.* Most people already know that caffeine and sleep don't mix (if I have caffeine at ten in the morning, I have trouble sleeping at night), but fewer people realize that alcohol can impair sleep. According to WebMD, studies show that alcohol ingestion impairs sleep quality, disrupting restorative REM (rapid eye movement) sleep.

- *Don't use screens for at least two hours before bedtime.* Research reported in *Scientific American* notes that people using backlit LED screens two hours or fewer before bedtime suffer impaired sleep due to disruptions in circadian rhythms. These screens might include tablets, laptop computers, and smartphones, among others.

Along with the above recommendations from the CDC, the National Sleep Foundation also recommends:

- *Don't nap during the day*, because it can cause disrupted sleep at night. I have found that even a 15-minute daytime nap really screws up my ability to sleep at night, which makes me sad, because I love naps.

- *If possible, get regular exercise.* Regular exercise before about 3 p.m. is especially helpful in promoting a good night's sleep. If you exercise at night, try a relaxing exercise like yoga or gentle stretching.

- *Use your bed only for sleep.* Don't read, eat, or watch television in bed. Instead, make your bed the place you sleep.

- *Get daily exposure to natural light.* Remember from our vitamin D discussion, all you need is 10 to 15 minutes to help set your body's circadian rhythms and allow you to sleep on a more natural sleep-wake cycle.

Sleep Disorders

If you are practicing good sleep hygiene and getting the recommended eight hours but are still waking unrefreshed, you may have an underlying sleep disorder, such as sleep apnea or restless leg syndrome (RLS). Talk with your doctor about possible sleep disorders; he or she may order a sleep study to determine whether there are other sleep-related issues and prescribe action.

Throughout the four-week plan, you will find specific suggestions to help you improve your sleep hygiene.

CHAPTER 4 TO-DOS

- Be aware of your mind-body connection. Journal about how your mind feels on days when you are feeling good physically; pay attention to how your body starts to feel when your mind is cluttered. Educate yourself more on this powerful connection and learn to bridge the gap between your mind and body. Your Hashimoto's will be relieved in ways that will astound you.

- Adopt a stress-relieving activity you can engage in when you're feeling stressed.

- Pay attention to the words your inner critic speaks to you. As you notice your inner critical voice, change harsh words to those of self-care and self-compassion.

- Review your sleep environment and make any necessary improvements to make it more comfortable and conducive to sleep.

- Turn off screens two hours before bedtime and don't bring your smartphone to bed.

- Devise a sleep plan. Determine the best time to go to sleep and wake up to get an optimal amount of sleep, and then arrange your day so you can stick to the plan.

- If you are waking up after a full night's sleep unrefreshed, talk to your doctor about the possibility of sleep disorders.

DAILY CHECK-IN

Pausing to check in with your body is helpful in tracking your health.

- Scan your body and notice any physical sensations.

- Turn your attention inward and notice any thoughts or feelings that come up.

- Remember that changes to your diet, stress levels, or rest can affect how you're feeling right now.

- Do something nice for yourself to cultivate feelings of well-being.

5

HEALING HASHIMOTO'S ON MULTIPLE FRONTS

Now we come to the nuts and bolts of the plan, where you will take specific action to bring about better health. Over the next four weeks, you will make changes in your eating habits and strive for better self-care. The goal is to begin integrating activities, habits, and knowledge into several areas of your life—mind, body, and spirit—to achieve a 360-degree view of your health. You deserve to feel well, and by committing to the next four weeks, you're taking important steps toward a lifetime of better health.

FOUR WEEKS, FOUR GOALS

During the next four weeks, you will be working toward improving your health on these multiple fronts:

1. Improving your diet and nutrition
2. Decreasing stress levels
3. Practicing more self-compassion
4. Improving sleep hygiene

You will not succeed if you do not make yourself a priority, starting right now. Set aside the time and energy to dedicate to planning grocery lists, soliciting support from friends and loved ones, and allotting 10 or 15 minutes per day for some peace and quiet. After the four weeks, you will be encouraged to continue the practices that you discovered work best for you so that you can continue to live a lifestyle that supports your overall health.

Making changes on multiple fronts over four weeks may sound intense, but this plan is designed to keep things simple for you. The food is delicious, and you will find the activities pleasurable and self-supportive.

Your Customized Recovery Plan

I've mentioned several times that this plan is designed to be customized to meet your specific needs. It's up to you to determine what works for you and what doesn't. However, I urge you to give each suggestion a long enough chance to see what truly works. Monitor yourself over the next four weeks by journaling and using the checklists and exercises throughout this book. Keep copious notes so you don't forget what works and what doesn't and what you'd like to share with your healthcare team.

Each week centers on four specific sections:

1. Elimination meal plan with specific recipes and shopping lists
2. Stress management techniques
3. Self-compassion practices
4. Sleep strategies

By the end of just one month's time, you will have participated in four different elimination meal plans, zeroing in on food sensitivities, inflammation foods, and even allergens. You'll also discover new foods and keep tabs on foods that make you feel terrific. Also, by the end of the month, you will have four helpful sleep strategies, self-compassion exercises, and ideas for stress management. Just think, 30 days is all it will take to start shifting your health in a positive direction! Do the Daily Check-In that appears throughout Part 1 to note how the strategies seem to be affecting your physical, mental, emotional, and spiritual wellness.

You are welcome to adapt or change strategies as needed depending on your needs and lifestyle. It's important that you work within your own capabilities and time constraints and don't push yourself too hard; it's okay to go to the edge, but don't go over it.

The Die-Off Reaction

In some cases, things might get slightly worse before they get better. As you change your habits, you may notice a slight uptick in symptoms, known as a die-off reaction, or the Jarisch-Herxheimer reaction. This reaction occurs when toxins in your system die off, most likely in response to a healthier, less toxic diet and healthier habits. As the toxins die, they release toxic byproducts into your system. As your body works to expel them, you may notice some symptoms for a few days.

While this may sound bad—toxins being released into your system—it's actually a good thing, because your body will excrete these by-products quickly enough, and you'll start to feel better. Plus, you'll no longer have the toxic organisms in your system.

To alleviate some of the die-off reactions:

- Drink plenty of filtered water to help flush the toxins out more quickly.
- Engage in gentle movement, which can help you sweat out toxins.
- Breathe deeply several times throughout the day to increase oxygen in the bloodstream.
- Get plenty of rest to support your body as it works to rid the toxins.

Making Room for My Needs

I t's easy to tell someone that they need to practice better self-care, but for many of us, following through can be tough. One major obstacle for many people is time—or lack of it.

Take a few minutes to think about your weekly schedule. Are there behaviors, tasks, or responsibilities that can be modified or removed? Jot down a few possibilities for each week, and then select one activity to modify or skip, giving you extra time in your schedule for critical self-care.

Week 1

1 *Skip 1 non-crucial errand this week.*

2 *Take bus and use that time to read.*

3 *Reschedule dinner with friends.*

THIS WEEK, I CHOOSE TO . . .

Reschedule dinner with friends. I'll see them next week instead.

Week 2

1 _____

2 _____

3 _____

THIS WEEK, I CHOOSE TO . . .

Week 3

1 _____

2 _____

3 _____

THIS WEEK, I CHOOSE TO . . .

Week 4

1 _____

2 _____

3 _____

THIS WEEK, I CHOOSE TO . . .

Week 1:
The Journey Begins

In the following pages, you'll find four weekly plans. Each week starts with a meal plan. Then you'll find self-care strategies for managing stress, practicing self-compassion, and improving your sleep. Alongside the strategies is a daily schedule where you can jot down self-care strategies you want to try for each day. Lastly, at the end of each week are explanations to help you implement the self-care strategies, as well as the weekly shopping list.

It is best if you have set yourself up for success ahead of time by cleaning your cupboards and refrigerator and stocking them with healthy foods, and setting aside time in your schedule for self-care. It is also important that before you begin week 1, you spend time explaining to your family what they might expect and asking for their support.

Monday

Breakfast	Apple-Cinnamon Oatmeal (page 133)
Lunch	Lettuce Cups with Egg Salad (page 160)
Dinner	Ground Beef Soup with Caramelized Onions and Caraway (page 170)
Snacks	Zucchini Hummus (page 155), coconut yogurt with blueberries, handful of sunflower seeds

Tuesday

Breakfast	Pumpkin Pie Smoothie (page 145)
Lunch	Leftover Ground Beef Soup with Caramelized Onions and Caraway
Dinner	Sweet Potato, Shiitake, and Spinach Curry (page 173)
Snacks	Leftover Zucchini Hummus, apple, deli turkey meat

Wednesday

Breakfast	Easy Egg, Sausage, and Sweet Potato Casserole (page 142)
Lunch	Leftover Lettuce Cups with Egg Salad
Dinner	Turkey Burgers, Protein Style (page 191)
Snacks	Festive Fruit Salad (page 161), coconut yogurt with blueberries and 1 tablespoon flaxseed, leftover deli turkey meat

Thursday

Breakfast	Coconut Flour and Flaxseed Porridge (page 135)
Lunch	Pumpkin Soup with Sage (page 164)
Dinner	Asparagus Quiche (page 182)
Snacks	Leftover Festive Fruit Salad, leftover Zucchini Hummus, carrot sticks with sunflower butter

Friday

Breakfast	Leftover Easy Egg, Sausage, and Sweet Potato Casserole
Lunch	Leftover Asparagus Quiche
Dinner	Asian Pork Meatballs with Gingered Bok Choy (page 202)
Snacks	Deli turkey meat, hard-boiled egg, pear

Saturday

Breakfast	Mushroom Frittata (page 141)
Lunch	Garlic and Spinach Zucchini Ribbons (page 174)
Dinner	Pan-Seared Pork Chops with Apple Butter (page 200)
Snacks	Leftover Apple Butter and carrot sticks, handful of sunflower seeds, Jicama and Avocado Dip (page 153)

Sunday

Breakfast	Pumpkin Waffles (page 139) with Apple Butter (page 225)
Lunch	Leftover Mushroom Frittata
Dinner	Easy Roast Chicken with Root Vegetables (page 190)
Snacks	Leftover Jicama and Avocado Dip, plain coconut yogurt with Apple Butter (page 225), Easy Sweet Potato Fries (page 154)

Self-Care Schedule

For each day of the week, choose a strategy from each of the following sections or create your own. Use the blank schedule to help you keep track of your choices.

Stress Management

1. Practice five minutes (or more) of gentle, repetitive movement.
2. Ask family members to help you with one task.
3. Simplify your schedule.

Self-Compassion

1. Commit to spending 15 minutes connecting with someone you love.
2. Practice mindful eating.
3. Write a note to yourself listing positive things about you.

Sleep Hygiene

1. Shut off all screens at least an hour before bedtime.
2. Go to bed 30 minutes earlier.
3. Use a white noise generator while you sleep.

Monday

Stress Management _____

Self-Compassion _____

Sleep Hygiene _____

Tuesday

Stress Management _____

Self-Compassion _____

Sleep Hygiene _____

Wednesday

Stress Management _____

Self-Compassion _____

Sleep Hygiene _____

Thursday

Stress Management _____

Self-Compassion _____

Sleep Hygiene _____

Friday

Stress Management _____

Self-Compassion _____

Sleep Hygiene _____

Saturday

Stress Management _____

Self-Compassion _____

Sleep Hygiene _____

Sunday

Stress Management _____

Self-Compassion _____

Sleep Hygiene _____

1

Stress Management

Practice five minutes (or more) of gentle repetitive movement. Also known as "movement meditation," this can be done while walking, riding an exercise cycle, tai chi, or any other gentle repetitive movement. Breathe deeply and clear your mind as you go through the movements. Try not to focus on anything other than movement and the present moment.

Ask family members to help you with one task. Each family member can choose a simple task you normally do, such as washing dishes or folding laundry, to give you more time to rest and care for yourself.

Simplify your schedule. If you have a lengthy to-do list, commit to only three or four items on that list, and be okay with completing only those. The rest can wait.

Self-Compassion

Commit to spending 15 minutes connecting with someone you love. Whether it's a quiet conversation, some simple cuddle time, or a phone call in the afternoon, connecting to people helps us feel good. It can be anyone who is a positive force to be around (even a pet).

Practice mindful eating. Set aside time for at least one meal or snack where you don't engage in any other activity except for the sensations associated with eating (in other words, no TV, no computer, no books—just silence and eating). Pay attention to how the food smells, tastes, and feels.

Write a note to yourself listing positive things about you. Tell yourself the things you'd love to hear someone else say to you. Take the time to read your notes to yourself each day.

Sleep Hygiene

Shut off all screens at least one hour before bedtime. Instead, read a book. You can also install a free app like flux (justgetflux.com) to help manage screen brightness throughout the day so it doesn't disrupt circadian rhythms.

Go to bed 30 minutes earlier. Even 30 minutes of extra sleep can make a big difference. Ideally, your goal is to adjust your sleep time per night to seven to eight hours.

Use a white noise generator while you sleep. A white noise-generating app cancels out noise, helping you get more restful sleep. Consider using a free app on your computer, tablet, or smartphone. I like the Brainwave app by Banzai Labs (banzailabs.com/brainwaveapps.html).

Week 1 Shopping List

FRUITS & VEGETABLES

Apples, 14
Asparagus, 1 bunch
Avocados, 2
Blueberries, 1 pint
Bok choy, 1 head
Carrots, 6 large
Grapes, 1 pound
Jicama, 1
Lemon, 1
Lettuce (iceberg),
  1 head
Lime, 1
Melon (honeydew), 1
Mushrooms (cremini),
  8 ounces
Mushrooms (shiitake),
  1 pound
Onions (red), 1
Onions (yellow), 7
Peaches, 2
Pear, 1
Scallions, 1 bunch
Shallots, 9
Spinach (baby),
  12 ounces
Strawberries, 1 pint
Sweet potato, 6
Zucchini, 4

HERBS & SPICES

Basil, 1 large bunch
Caraway, ground
Chives, 1 bunch
Cilantro, 1 bunch
Cloves, ground
Cinnamon, ground
Cumin, ground
Curry paste, red
Garlic, 2 bulbs
Ginger, 1 knob
Mustard powder, dried
Nutmeg, 1
Rosemary, dried
Sage, ground
Tarragon (fresh), 1 bunch
Thyme, dried
Turmeric, ground
Vanilla extract

MEAT & EGGS

Beef (ground), 1 pound
Chicken (whole roaster),
  5 to 6 pounds
Eggs, 3 dozen
Pork (boneless,
  thick-cut chops), 4
Pork (ground), 2 pounds
Turkey (deli slices),
  1 pound
Turkey (ground), 1 pound

CANNED

Coconut milk,
  2 (14-ounce) cans
Pumpkin purée
  (unsweetened),
  1 (15-ounce) can and
  1 (29-ounce) can

OILS

Avocado oil (cold-pressed)
Coconut oil (cold-pressed)
Olive oil (extra-virgin)

DAIRY

Yogurt (coconut, plain),
  2 large containers

SEEDS

Flaxseed, 4 ounces
Sunflower seeds (raw),
  about 1 cup

OTHER

Apple cider vinegar
Baking powder
Beef broth, 1 (48-ounce)
  carton
Chicken broth, 1 cup
Coconut flour
Fish sauce
Nutritional yeast
Oats, steel cut, 2 cups
Rice milk (plain), 4 cups
Soy sauce or tamari
  (gluten-free)
Stevia, liquid
Tahini
Tapioca flour
Vegetable broth,
  1 (24-ounce) carton
Worcestershire sauce

Week 2:
Adjusting to a New Lifestyle

You have been adjusting to your new lifestyle changes, and by the end of week 1, hopefully you are feeling a bit more well rested and in control. Likewise, your body is adapting to a greater state of nourishment. If you experienced any die-off recovery symptoms, some may still be lingering, but they should be about gone. As you go through week 2, think of how you can adapt habits to make your cooking requirements easier, such as cooking ahead and freezing foods, or cooking more than you need and eating leftovers.

Consider giving your family a progress report and sharing with them the changes you plan to make this week. Don't forget to check in with yourself using the Daily Check-In throughout part 1, listening to your body, and recording how you feel.

Monday

Breakfast	Slow Cooker Breakfast Rice (page 134)
Lunch	Leftover Easy Roast Chicken with green salad and Basil Vinaigrette (page 230)
Dinner	Tri-Tip Tacos (page 204)
Snacks	Coconut Gelatin (page 149), hard-boiled egg, plain coconut yogurt with sunflower seeds and chopped apple

Tuesday

Breakfast	Mixed Berry–Chia Smoothie (page 151)
Lunch	Mushroom Soup (page 166)
Dinner	Ground Beef and Asparagus Stir-Fry (page 207)
Snacks	Leftover Coconut Gelatin, apple slices with sunflower butter, carrot sticks

Wednesday

Breakfast	Leftover Slow Cooker Breakfast Rice
Lunch	Veggie and Rice Stir-Fry (page 176)
Dinner	Turkey and Spinach Roulade (page 192)
Snacks	Hard-boiled egg, carrot sticks and sunflower butter, Simple Green Smoothie (page 146)

Thursday

Breakfast	Easy Banana Pancakes (page 138) with Apple Butter (page 225)
Lunch	Leftover Mushroom Soup
Dinner	Slow Cooker Beef Stew with Fennel and Mushrooms (page 205)
Snacks	Apple Butter and celery sticks, Cucumber Salad with Ginger-Cilantro Vinaigrette (page 157), Avocado-Garlic Deviled Eggs (page 152)

Friday

Breakfast	Sautéed Spinach with Fried Eggs (page 186)
Lunch	Leftover Veggie and Rice Stir-Fry
Dinner	Bacon-Wrapped Drumsticks with Asparagus (page 196)
Snacks	Banana and sunflower seeds, apple, celery sticks and carrot sticks

Saturday

Breakfast	Coconut Flour Pancakes with Berries (page 136)
Lunch	Leftover Bacon-Wrapped Drumsticks with Asparagus
Dinner	Gyro Salad (page 208)
Snacks	Leftover Cucumber Salad with Ginger-Cilantro Vinaigrette, Leftover Avocado-Garlic Deviled Eggs, plain coconut yogurt with Apple Butter (page 225)

Sunday

Breakfast	Bacon Cups with Baked Eggs (page 143)
Lunch	Sweet Potato Hash Browns with Sautéed Mushrooms (page 184)
Dinner	Herb-Rubbed Leg of Lamb (page 209)
Snacks	Prosciutto-wrapped honeydew melon, carrot sticks, handful of sunflower seeds

2

Self-Care Schedule

For each day of the week, choose a strategy from each of the following sections or create your own. Use the blank schedule to help you keep track of your choices.

Stress Management

1. Practice saying no to the many requests people bring to you.
2. In the shower, practice gentle neck and upper back stretches.
3. Spend a few minutes each day cleaning out a messy drawer.

Self-Compassion

1. Try to make a connection with people you meet in passing.
2. Spend a few minutes in nature noticing the beauty all around you.
3. Practice a daily affirmation about something you'd like to achieve or feel.

Sleep Hygiene

1. Keep an aromatherapy scent that promotes sleep in your bedroom.
2. Try to get as much natural light as you can throughout the day.
3. Make your bed strictly a place to sleep.

Monday

Stress Management _____

Self-Compassion _____

Sleep Hygiene _____

Tuesday

Stress Management _____

Self-Compassion _____

Sleep Hygiene _____

Wednesday

Stress Management _____

Self-Compassion _____

Sleep Hygiene _____

Thursday

Stress Management _____

Self-Compassion _____

Sleep Hygiene _____

Friday

Stress Management _____

Self-Compassion _____

Sleep Hygiene _____

Saturday

Stress Management _____

Self-Compassion _____

Sleep Hygiene _____

Sunday

Stress Management _____

Self-Compassion _____

Sleep Hygiene _____

2

Stress Management

Practice saying no to the many requests people bring to you. Instead, say yes only to those tasks and activities in which you really want to engage.

In the shower, practice gentle neck and upper back stretches. Put your chin to your chest and gently roll across your chest, taking your ear to each shoulder. Shrug your shoulders up and down. Turn your chin to your left and right shoulders. The hot water will make these stretches comfortable and help in easing tension.

Spend a few minutes each day cleaning out a messy drawer. You know you have one (or more) drawers or closets that totally stress you out. Instead of undertaking a massive cleaning project, focus on working on one at a time, just organizing for about five minutes a day.

Self-Compassion

Try to make a connection with people you meet in passing. It doesn't have to be a "suddenly their eyes met across the room" type of connection. It can just be a friendly smile or a kind word.

Spend a few minutes in nature noticing the beauty all around you. Notice the fresh clean smell of the air. Listen to the sound of birds or rain. Feel the breeze lightly ruffle your hair. Notice how solid the earth is underneath your feet.

Practice a daily affirmation about something you'd like to achieve or feel. It can be something simple, such as "I am surrounded by love," or it can be very specific, such as, "Today I am filled with energy." Make your affirmation as a positive statement. Repeat it five times each day.

Sleep Hygiene

Keep an aromatherapy scent that promotes sleep in your bedroom. A diffuser is a great way to distribute scent in the bedroom, although it can be as simple as a few drops on a cotton ball next to the bed. Sleep-promoting scents include lavender, chamomile, and special sleep blends.

Try to get as much natural light as you can throughout the day. Go outdoors when you can, or spend time near a window. Keep your curtains and blinds open during the day to allow as much natural light as possible to pour through them.

Make your bed strictly a place to sleep. Don't eat there, watch television, listen to the radio, or hang out with family. Banish pets from your bed, too. If you read before bed, do it in a comfy chair in your bedroom or in the living room.

Week 2 Shopping List

FRUITS & VEGETABLES

Apples, 9

Arugula, 2 bunches

Asparagus, 3 bunches

Avocados, 3

Bananas, 3

Carrots, 6

Celery, 1 bunch

Cucumbers, 2

Fennel, 1 bulb

Leek, 1

Lemon, 1

Lettuce (romaine),
  2 heads

Lime, 1

Melon (honeydew), 1

Mushrooms (cremini),
  3 pounds

Mushrooms (porcini,
  dried), 4 ounces

Mushrooms (shiitake),
  1 pound

Onions (red), 3

Onion (yellow), 1

Orange, 1

Raspberries, 1 pint

Scallions, 3 bunches

Shallots, 2

Spinach (baby),
  2 pounds

Sweet potatoes, 2

HERBS & SPICES

Basil, 2 bunches

Chives, 1 bunch

Cilantro, 1 bunch

Cinnamon, ground

Cloves, ground

Garlic, 3 bulbs

Ginger, 1 knob

Rosemary (fresh),
  1 bunch

Vanilla extract
  (alcohol-free, pure)

MEAT & EGGS

Bacon (thin-sliced),
  2 pounds

Beef (ground), 1 pound

Beef (tri-tip), 1½ pounds

Beef (stewing meat),
  1½ pounds

Chicken
  (drumsticks), 12

Eggs, 3 dozen

Lamb (ground),
  2 pounds

Lamb (leg), 5 pounds

Pancetta, 4 ounces

Prosciutto (sliced),
  4 ounces

Turkey (boneless
  breast), 1 pound

CANNED

Coconut milk (lite),
  5 (14-ounce) cans

FROZEN

Berries (mixed), 2 cups

Blueberries, 1 cup

Blackberries, ½ cup

DAIRY

Yogurt (coconut, plain),
  2 large containers

SEEDS

Chia seeds, 4 ounces

Sunflower seeds (raw),
  about 1 cup

OTHER

Apple juice (unsweetened),
  16 ounces

Apricots (dried), ½ cup

Arrowroot powder

Chicken broth,
  1 (32-ounce) carton

Gelatin

Mustard, Dijon

Raisins, ½ cup

Red wine vinegar

Rice, brown

Rice milk (plain,
  unsweetened), 2 cups

Rice, precooked brown,
  2 cups

2

Week 3:
Hitting Your Stride

By now, you're well into your program. Hopefully you're seeing positive changes, noticing diminishing symptoms, and feeling well rested and less stressed. This is a good time to go back and review any changes in your symptoms, because sometimes they can be subtle. I know that if I don't write symptoms down, I often forget they even existed once they've been gone a while. This week the Daily Check-In is of special importance because you will likely notice progress now. It can be quite motivating to see tangible, trackable changes, and to realize that things are getting better, even if in subtle ways.

Monday

Breakfast	Leftover Bacon Cups with Baked Eggs
Lunch	Leftover Gyro Salad
Dinner	Minted Quinoa and Vegetables (page 177)
Snacks	Jicama and Avocado Dip (page 153), hard-boiled egg, apple

Tuesday

Breakfast	Piña Colada Smoothie (page 148)
Lunch	Leftover Herb-Rubbed Leg of Lamb and green salad with Basil Vinaigrette (page 230)
Dinner	Pork Tenderloin with Onions, Figs, and Rosemary (page 198)
Snacks	Prosciutto-wrapped honeydew melon, grapes with plain coconut yogurt, celery sticks with sunflower butter

Wednesday

Breakfast	Easy Egg, Sausage, and Sweet Potato Casserole (page 142)
Lunch	Leftover Minted Quinoa and Vegetables
Dinner	Pot Roast with Sweet Potato and Shallots (page 206)
Snacks	Leftover Jicama and Avocado Dip, Festive Fruit Salad (page 161), half of a baked sweet potato

Thursday

Breakfast	Pumpkin Pie Smoothie (page 145)
Lunch	Pesto Zoodles (page 183)
Dinner	Turkey and Spinach Roulade (page 192)
Snacks	Leftover Festive Fruit Salad, hard-boiled egg, carrot sticks with sunflower butter

Friday

Breakfast	Leftover Easy Egg, Sausage, and Sweet Potato Casserole
Lunch	Leftover Pork Tenderloin with Onions, Figs, and Rosemary
Dinner	Turkey Burgers, Protein Style (page 191)
Snacks	Leftover half of a baked sweet potato, Guacamole (page 234) and carrot sticks, plain coconut yogurt with leftover Festive Fruit Salad

Saturday

Breakfast	Mushroom Frittata (page 141)
Lunch	Leftover Pesto Zoodles
Dinner	Asian Pork Meatballs with Gingered Bok Choy (page 202)
Snacks	Pear, handful of sunflower seeds, Easy Sweet Potato Fries (page 154)

Sunday

Breakfast	Coconut Flour Pancakes with Berries (page 136)
Lunch	Leftover Pot Roast with Sweet Potatoes and Shallots
Dinner	Slow Cooker Chicken and Mushroom Stew (page 189)
Snacks	Leftover Guacamole and celery sticks, plain coconut yogurt with blueberries and sunflower seeds, deli turkey meat

Self-Care Schedule

For each day of the week, choose a strategy from each of the following sections or create your own. Use the blank schedule to help you keep track of your choices.

Stress Management

1. Make a list of all you do and pare it down to only the important things.
2. Use progressive relaxation at night before going to sleep.
3. When you are feeling anxious, say to yourself, "Let it go."

Self-Compassion

1. Choose one person and tell them why you appreciate them.
2. Spend five to ten minutes in meditative activity.
3. Practice some positive self-talk.

Sleep Hygiene

1. Remove light pollution from your sleep environment.
2. Stick to your bedtime and wake-up time.
3. Stop eating/drinking at least an hour before bedtime.

Monday

Stress Management _____

Self-Compassion _____

Sleep Hygiene _____

Tuesday

Stress Management _____

Self-Compassion _____

Sleep Hygiene _____

Wednesday

Stress Management _____

Self-Compassion _____

Sleep Hygiene _____

Thursday

Stress Management _____

Self-Compassion _____

Sleep Hygiene _____

Friday

Stress Management _____

Self-Compassion _____

Sleep Hygiene _____

Saturday

Stress Management _____

Self-Compassion _____

Sleep Hygiene _____

Sunday

Stress Management _____

Self-Compassion _____

Sleep Hygiene _____

3

Stress Management

Make a list of all you do and pare it down to only the important things. There's a lot of nonessential busy-ness and noise in most people's lives. Take an objective look at your to-do lists. What is essential? Keep those things on the list and discard the rest.

Use progressive relaxation at night before going to sleep. Close your eyes and, starting at your feet, relax your entire body, one muscle at a time. If you're a person who ruminates, this one is for you.

When you are feeling anxious, say to yourself, "Let it go." Notice when your anxiety is ramping up. When you start to feel the telltale signs of anxiety, close your eyes, breathe deeply, and repeat to yourself, "Let it go."

Self-Compassion

Choose one person and tell them why you appreciate them. Social media makes this activity especially easy, but you don't need it to do it. Being kind to others makes you feel really good about yourself, and it is usually contagious.

Spend five to ten minutes in meditative activity. While this could be meditation (such as sitting quietly and speaking a mantra), meditative activity can be any activity you enjoy that takes you out of your brain. Try reading, listening to music, deep breathing, or engaging in a hobby you love.

Practice some positive self-talk. Forgiving yourself when you make a mistake or praising yourself when you succeed is necessary to keep you on the path to wellness.

Sleep Hygiene

Remove light pollution from your sleep environment. Light in your bedroom can mess up the quality and quantity of your sleep, so it's to your benefit to make your room as dark as possible. If you can't sufficiently darken your environment, then use a sleep mask.

Stick to your bedtime and wake-up time. One of the best ways to set your body clock for sleep is to go to bed and wake up at the same time every night and morning, even on the weekends. Optimally, you should try for seven to eight hours of sleep each night.

Stop eating and drinking at least an hour before bedtime. Eating too close to bed is disruptive to sleep. Also don't drink liquids before bedtime to keep from getting up at night.

Week 3 Shopping List

FRUITS & VEGETABLES

Apples, 2
Avocados, 2
Bok choy, 1 head
Carrots, 6
Celery, 1 bunch
Fennel, 1 bulb
Figs, 10
Grapes, 1 pound
Jicama, 1
Lemon, 1
Lettuce (iceberg),
  1 head
Lime, 1
Melon (honeydew), 1
Mushrooms (cremini),
  1½ pound
Mushrooms (shiitake),
  8 ounces
Onion (red), 1
Onions (yellow), 5
Peaches, 2
Pear, 1
Pineapple chunks,
  2 cups
Scallions, 1 bunch
Shallots, 6
Spinach (baby),
  1½ pounds
Strawberries, 1 pint
Sweet potatoes, 6
Zucchini, 4

HERBS & SPICES

Basil, 2 bunches
Chives, 1 bunch
Cilantro, 1 bunch
Garlic, 2 bulbs
Garlic powder
Ginger, 1 knob
Mint, 1 bunch
Nutmeg, ground
Rum extract

MEAT & EGGS

Beef (chuck roast),
  3 pounds
Chicken (bone-in,
  skin-on thighs), 8
Eggs, 3 dozen
Pork (ground), 2 pounds
Pork (tenderloin),
  2 pounds
Turkey (boneless
  breast), 1 pound
Turkey (deli slices),
  1 pound
Turkey (ground),
  1 pound

CANNED

Coconut milk,
  3 (14-ounce) cans
Coconut milk (lite),
  3 (14-ounce) cans
Pumpkin purée
  (pure unsweetened),
  1 (15-ounce) can

FROZEN

Blueberries, 1 cup
Blackberries, ½ cup

DAIRY

Yogurt (coconut, plain),
  2 large containers

SEEDS

Pumpkin seeds (raw),
  1½ cups

OTHER

Apple juice (unsweetened),
  8 ounces
Balsamic vinegar
Beef broth, 1 (32-ounce)
  carton
Chicken broth, 2 cups
Quinoa
Rice milk (plain,
  unsweetened), ¼ cup
Vegetable broth, 2 cups

Week 4:
Celebrating Your Progress

4

You've made it to week 4. Congratulations on making healthier choices and caring deeply for yourself! While this is the last official week of the plan, I hope you will be able to find enough ideas that make a true difference in how you feel. Although I've suggested you try only one of each type of activity per week, in the weeks that follow, feel free to go back and implement other suggestions to see if they work for you as well. Ultimately, the goal is for you to find a plan of action that works best for you.

Monday

Breakfast	Apple-Cinnamon Oatmeal (page 133)
Lunch	Leftover Mushroom Frittata
Dinner	Stuffed Zucchini Boats (page 180)
Snacks	Deli turkey meat, Piña Colada Smoothie (page 148), handful of sunflower seeds

Tuesday

Breakfast	Mixed Berry-Chia Smoothie (page 151)
Lunch	Leftover Slow Cooker Chicken and Mushroom Stew
Dinner	Asparagus Quiche (page 182)
Snacks	Prosciutto-wrapped asparagus, sliced cantaloupe, Avocado-Garlic Deviled Eggs (page 152)

Wednesday

Breakfast	Coconut Flour and Flaxseed Porridge (page 135)
Lunch	Leftover Asparagus Quiche
Dinner	Pan-Seared Pork Chops with Apple Butter (page 200)
Snacks	Zucchini Hummus (page 155) and carrot sticks, deli turkey meat-wrapped asparagus, pear

Thursday

Breakfast	Easy Banana Pancakes (page 138) with Apple Butter (page 225)
Lunch	Ground Beef Soup with Caramelized Onions and Caraway (page 170)
Dinner	Gyro Salad (page 208)
Snacks	Plain coconut yogurt with Apple Butter, leftover Avocado-Garlic Deviled Eggs, deli turkey meat

Friday

Breakfast	Pumpkin Waffles (page 139)
Lunch	Leftover Gyro Salad
Dinner	Bacon-Wrapped Drumsticks with Asparagus (page 196)
Snacks	Leftover Zucchini Hummus and carrot sticks, pear slices and sunflower butter, celery sticks

Saturday

Breakfast	Sautéed Spinach with Fried Eggs (page 186)
Lunch	Leftover Ground Beef Soup with Caramelized Onions and Caraway
Dinner	Cobb Salad (page 158) with Basil Vinaigrette (page 230)
Snacks	Deli turkey meat, Coconut Gelatin (page 149), Easy Sweet Potato Fries (page 154)

Sunday

Breakfast	Bacon Cups with Baked Eggs (page 143)
Lunch	Leftover Bacon-Wrapped Drumsticks with Asparagus
Dinner	Easy Roast Chicken with Root Vegetables (page 190)
Snacks	Leftover Coconut Gelatin, Simple Green Smoothie (page 146), unsweetened applesauce

4

Self-Care Schedule

For each day of the week, choose a strategy from each of the following sections or create your own. Use the blank schedule to help you keep track of your choices.

Stress Management

1. Practice not justifying your choices to anyone else.
2. Get up and move throughout the day.
3. Examine what frightens you.

Self-Compassion

1. Pay it forward.
2. Do chores more mindfully.
3. Practice gratitude.

Sleep Hygiene

1. Make time for sleep.
2. Cut out stimulants.
3. Adjust your room temperature.

Monday

Stress Management _____

Self-Compassion _____

Sleep Hygiene _____

Tuesday

Stress Management _____

Self-Compassion _____

Sleep Hygiene _____

Wednesday

Stress Management _____

Self-Compassion _____

Sleep Hygiene _____

Thursday

Stress Management _____

Self-Compassion _____

Sleep Hygiene _____

Friday

Stress Management _____

Self-Compassion _____

Sleep Hygiene _____

Saturday

Stress Management _____

Self-Compassion _____

Sleep Hygiene _____

Sunday

Stress Management _____

Self-Compassion _____

Sleep Hygiene _____

4

Stress Management

Practice not justifying your choices to anyone else. This week, when you tell people no, do it with a smile and no explanation. If they demand an explanation, just say no once again.

Get up and move throughout the day. This is especially important if you have a sitting job. Every hour or so, take a few minutes to stand up and stroll around or, at the very least, stretch and move a little.

Examine what frightens you. This week, try to catch yourself thinking stress-inducing or fearful thoughts and take a moment to think, "Why does this really scare me?"

Self-Compassion

Pay it forward. Making an effort to help others, even in tiny ways, can make your life so much more rewarding. These don't need to be grand gestures or large donations to charity, but can be something as simple as holding a door for someone or lending a compassionate ear.

Do chores more mindfully. Chores are only a drag if you make them so. If you do them mindfully, they can become a meditative exercise.

Practice gratitude. Even with a chronic illness, there is so much around for which to be grateful. On super bad days, that gratitude may be something basic like, "I'm grateful for air" or "I give thanks that my legs go all the way to the floor." But even in the darkest of times, there are gifts in your life.

Sleep Hygiene

Make time for sleep. If you have to watch your television shows, there's a way to get your shows and still go to sleep at a reasonable hour—things like DVR, Hulu, and Netflix. Make getting sleep a priority and work other activities around your sleep schedule.

Cut out stimulants. While this diet tries to do that by eliminating sugar and caffeine, some people think they can't function without it, so they slip it in anyway. If you must continue with your caffeine, don't have any in the afternoon, so it won't disrupt your sleep.

Adjust your room temperature. Being too hot or too cold while you sleep can cause you to wake throughout the night. A humidifier in the room can also help to ease any breathing difficulties due to cold or dry air.

Week 4 Shopping List

FRUITS & VEGETABLES

Apples, 13
Arugula, 3 small bunches
Asparagus, 3 bunches
Avocados, 4
Bananas, 2
Cantaloupe, 1
Carrots, 6
Lemon, 1
Lettuce (romaine),
  1 head
Melon (honeydew), 1
Mushrooms (cremini),
  8 ounces
Onion (red), 1
Onions (yellow), 4
Orange, 1
Pears, 2
Pineapple chunks,
  2 cups
Raspberries, 1 pint
Scallions, 1 bunch
Shallots, 10
Spinach (baby), 1 pound
Strawberries, 1 pint
Sweet potatoes, 3
Zucchini, 5

HERBS & SPICES

Basil, 1 bunch
Chives, 1 bunch
Garlic, 3 bulbs
Ginger, 1 knob

MEAT & EGGS

Bacon (thin-sliced),
  2 pounds
Beef (ground), 1 pound
Chicken (drumsticks), 12
Chicken (rotisserie,
  cooked), 1
Chicken (whole roaster)
  5 to 6 pounds
Eggs, 4 dozen
Lamb (ground), 2 pounds
Pork (boneless, thick-cut
  chops), 4
Prosciutto, 8 ounces

CANNED

Coconut milk,
  3 (14-ounce) cans
Coconut milk (lite),
  5 (14-ounce) cans
Pumpkin purée
  (pure, unsweetened),
  1 (15-ounce) can

FROZEN

Berries (mixed), 2 cups

DAIRY

Yogurt (coconut, plain),
  2 large containers

OTHER

Apple juice (unsweetened),
  8 ounces
Applesauce (unsweetened),
  1 container
Beef broth, 1 (48-ounce)
  carton
Chicken broth, 1 cup
Gelatin
Oats, steel cut, 2 cups
Rice milk (plain,
  unsweetened), 1 cup
Tapioca flour
Vegetable broth,
  1 (32-ounce) carton

CLOSING THOUGHTS

Congratulations! You made it through the four-week program, hopefully with some great results. Now it's up to you to decide which of these activities work for you and which might require adjustment.

I used to be an all-or-nothing kind of gal, but I discovered that type of rigid thinking kept me from living my best life. Now I'm what I refer to as a 95 percenter: I follow my plan about 95 percent of the time, and the other 5 percent, I stray here and there. Although I've also learned which habits are deal breakers, from which I can never stray (such as eating gluten, which makes me very ill), I continuously try new things, observing how I feel and making adjustments. That's because sometimes things that used to work stop working so well, and sometimes I just need to try something new.

Your body is always changing, and you need to adapt. Flexibility is essential in dealing with a chronic illness like Hashimoto's, as is always making the kindest and most supportive choice for yourself. On the days you don't feel as well, be kinder to yourself. Rest. Relax. Eat well. On the days you feel terrific, try a little more. Let your body and your inner voice be your guides.

As you move beyond your four weeks, flexibility is key. It's up to you to always keep your own best interests at heart, monitoring your symptoms, listening to your inner guidance, and making adjustments as needed. Sometimes life gets in the way, and that's okay, too. Live the life you need, maintaining as many of your healthy habits as make sense in the moment, and then picking up more of them again once things return to normal.

I'd also like to make a gentle suggestion here about "falling off the wagon." We all do it. Sometimes you just feel like you want to drink that whole bottle of Champagne (and pay for it the next morning) or eat a candy bar. I get that. What's important here is not that you "fell" (or just slipped a little), but that you got back up and continued on your program, because you realize that ultimately, you are worth it, your health is important, and you deserve to live a fulfilling, healthy, and beautiful life.

CHAPTER 5 TO-DOS

☐ After the four weeks, begin reintroducing foods as you see fit (and as outlined), and determine which are triggers for you and which are fine.

☐ Plan your weeks ahead of time, choosing the activities that most appeal to you or those that seem the most beneficial.

☐ After the four weeks, go back and try some of the other strategies you ignored.

☐ Make an appointment with your doctor to discuss your health as you continue forward after the four weeks.

☐ Choose which habits you will maintain, new habits you'd like to try, and those that don't seem to benefit you.

☐ Continue recording your symptoms and checking in with your inner guidance as you move forward in order to adapt the plan to one that best suits your lifestyle.

☐ Give yourself credit for taking control of your life and your health and being far better off for it.

DAILY CHECK-IN

Pausing to check in with your body is helpful in tracking your health.

☐ Scan your body and notice any physical sensations.

☐ Turn your attention inward and notice any thoughts or feelings that come up.

☐ Remember that changes to your diet, stress levels, or rest can affect how you're feeling right now.

☐ Do something nice for yourself to cultivate feelings of well-being.

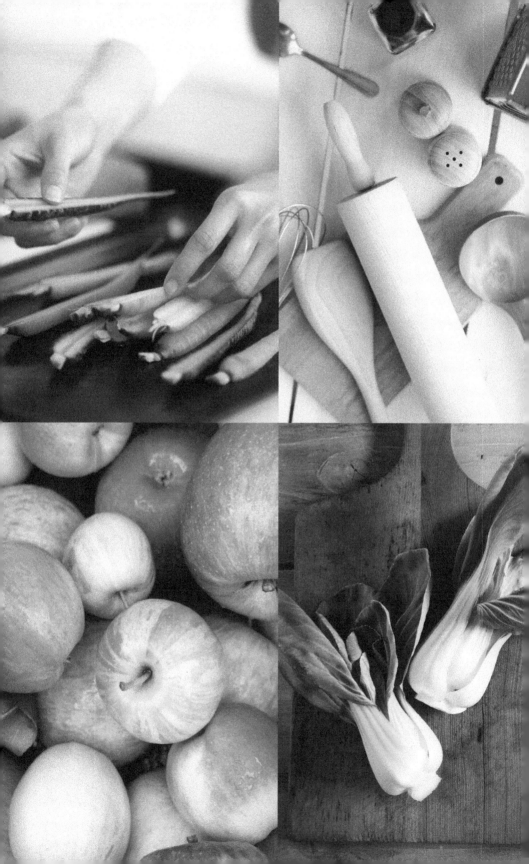

PART 2

Preparing Delicious Recipes

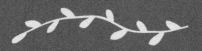

6

THE HASHIMOTO'S-FRIENDLY KITCHEN

Changing the way you eat requires preparation, and it begins in your kitchen. The recipes in the chapters that follow use everyday ingredients and do not require special equipment. Even so, it is a good idea to make certain that you have a pantry stocked with the foods you will need, as well as the kitchen equipment that makes preparation easy.

As a first step, go through your pantry and refrigerator shelves and your cupboards and, if possible, remove any foods that might tempt you. Replace them with the healthy foods that you will be using in your recipes. This will set the stage for success as you move forward.

TIPS FOR EASING THE TRANSITION

If you have never done a lot of cooking or have relied on heavily processed foods, then transitioning to a plan that requires more cooking might seem daunting. Keep these tips in mind as you begin your new plan.

Cook Once, Eat Twice

This is advice that I offer in all my cookbooks—and that I actually follow: With my dietary challenges, I very seldom eat food from restaurants, and I don't eat processed foods. I make virtually everything from scratch, which takes time. That's why I follow this tenet—*cook once, eat twice*. I prepare large batches so I get two or more meals out of each.

Your Freezer Is Your Friend

Sometimes I make batches that are large enough so I can also freeze leftovers. These frozen servings are my on-the-go foods. I pack them in a cooler when I travel and reheat them in the microwave. That way I am never stuck without a meal. Store the foods in microwave-safe freezer containers, labeled with the date you made the food and what it is.

Cook Ahead

If I have a busy week coming up, I will often prepare foods on the weekend and portion them out to be reheated as meals throughout the week. This is a great strategy for people with busy lives who don't have time to cook on weeknights.

Soup Is Good Food

I eat a lot of soup, especially during the colder months. Soup is wonderful because you can toss in some meat, veggies, herbs, and spices and have a simple, one-pot meal that comes together in a very short time. It also freezes and reheats very well, and it is a great food to feed your entire family. I make soup about once a week because it is such a great way to pack nourishing ingredients into a meal.

Learn to Love Your Slow Cooker

I believe that a slow cooker is an essential piece of kitchen equipment in busy households where you cook all the food you eat. With a slow cooker, you can toss in ingredients in the morning and come home to a hot, delicious meal.

Buy Prechopped Veggies

To save time, you can buy prechopped vegetables at the grocery store. You can also save time by using frozen vegetables for soups or stews.

ESSENTIAL EQUIPMENT

You do not need a lot of special equipment, but having some of the items that follow make food preparation and cooking a lot easier.

Blender, Immersion Blender, and/or Food Processor

Blending is a great way to thicken soups and stews without using a flour-based roux, heavy cream, or other thickeners. It's also helpful for making smoothies. You do not need all three of these; one will do the trick. The food processor is the most versatile since it can also chop veggies and herbs and perform a number of other functions, but a blender or immersion (stick) blender will also serve your purposes well for blending soups and smoothies.

Slow Cooker

A basic slow cooker is very affordable, and I believe it is essential equipment for the busy cook. I actually own four slow cookers in various sizes, but you don't need to get that enthusiastic about slow cooking. A large-capacity slow cooker (6 to 8 quarts) will work for any recipe in this book.

Spiralizer, Julienne Cutter, or Vegetable Peeler

To add texture and interest to your foods, and to help you not miss pasta so much, cutting zucchini and other vegetables into noodles is a delicious strategy. While a spiralizer is ideal for this purpose (and costs between $10 and $40), you can use simpler tools like a julienne cutter or a vegetable peeler and a sharp knife.

Sharp Knives

Many chefs consider their knives their most essential pieces of kitchen equipment, and so do I. Having a good-quality chef's knife and a high-quality paring knife will help you cut meat and produce safely and efficiently. Keeping blades in top condition with a knife sharpener is also necessary, because sharp knives are much safer than dull knives.

Oven-Safe Dutch Oven or Large Soup Pot with Lid

If you are making large batches, this is an essential piece of kitchen equipment. Cast iron is an excellent affordable alternative for this type of pot. Make sure it is free of plastic handles, since you may need to transfer it to the oven.

Pots and Pans

You will need several of these:

- Small, medium, and large saucepans
- Baking sheets
- Nonstick sauté pan
- Ovenproof sauté pan
- Baking pans: 9-inch square and 9-by-13-inch rectangular pan

Freezer to Microwave Storage Containers

You can find these glass or plastic containers at most grocery stores. Glass is nonreactive but more expensive, while there is some controversy about the potential health effects of plastic containers when you heat them in the microwave. I use both.

Meat Thermometer

The best way to tell if meat is done is to test it with a digital instant-read thermometer. You can find inexpensive thermometers at most kitchen supply stores and even some grocery stores.

Utensils

You will need a variety of utensils, including:

- Mixing spoons
- Rubber spatulas
- Spatulas
- Measuring cups (liquid and dry)
- Measuring spoons
- Whisks
- Graters (rasp style and box)
- Strainers (a fine-mesh sieve and an over- or in-the-sink colander)
- Cutting boards (you'll need two dishwasher-safe boards, one for meats and one for produce)

Mixing Bowls

Having a few sizes of mixing bowls is helpful. I really like the OXO Good Grips bowls because they have a handle, a pouring spout, and a rubberized bottom so they grip the counter when you are stirring, but any bowls will do. Get various sizes and have at least two or three.

Parchment Paper

Parchment paper is a convenient kitchen tool for lining baking sheets and pans or for cooking food, even a whole meal, in parchment packets.

STOCK YOUR PANTRY

Pantry items are those that you will use throughout the month in multiple recipes. They are shelf-stable or will last, opened, in the refrigerator or freezer for several weeks. These are the essential items that form the basis of many of the recipes.

Fats and Oils

- **Extra-virgin olive oil:** Don't purchase "lite" olive oil. And beware: some olive oils actually contain canola oil as well. My favorite 100 percent extra-virgin olive oil brand is California Olive Ranch, which is affordable and widely available in grocery stores.

- *Coconut oil:* Choose extra-virgin coconut oil, which is solid at room temperature. Choose organic if possible.
- *Avocado oil:* Choose organic, expeller-pressed.

Herbs and Spices

- *Sea salt or Himalayan pink salt:* Both have higher mineral content. I really love the pink salt, and I also enjoy Celtic sea salt. Choose a fine grain.
- *Black pepper:* While it's not necessary to freshly grind black pepper, I find the taste superior. If you have a pepper grinder, then choose black peppercorns. Otherwise, you can buy it already ground.
- *Cinnamon:* While it's a bit more expensive, look for ground Ceylon or Sri Lankan cinnamon, which is true cinnamon. Much of the ground cinnamon you find in the spice aisle is actually cassia.
- *Nutmeg:* If at all possible, buy whole nutmeg seeds and grate them with a rasp-style grater. Freshly grated nutmeg enhances the flavor of your dishes. Otherwise, go ahead and purchase it ground.
- *Dry mustard powder:* Check the label to make sure it doesn't contain any flour.
- *Vanilla extract:* Buy alcohol-free pure vanilla extract if you can find it, although you use such small amounts that the alcohol is not really a factor.

- *Cloves, ground*
- *Coriander, ground*
- *Cumin, ground*
- *Curry powder*
- *Garlic powder*
- *Ginger, ground*
- *Italian seasoning, dried*

- *Onion powder*
- *Oregano, dried*
- *Rosemary, dried*
- *Sage, dried*
- *Tarragon, dried*
- *Thyme, dried*
- *Turmeric, ground*

Canned Foods/Condiments

- **Coconut milk,** full-fat or lite
- **Pumpkin purée:** Choose a brand with only pumpkin as an ingredient. Don't accidentally buy pumpkin pie filling—it's not the same.
- **Red wine vinegar**
- **Apple cider vinegar:** Choose organic. My favorite brand is Bragg.
- **Dijon mustard:** Check the label to make sure it doesn't contain wheat flour. Grey Poupon is a good brand.
- **Gluten-free soy sauce or tamari:** Most tamari is gluten-free. Check the label.
- **Fish sauce:** My favorite brand is Red Boat.
- **Chicken, beef, or vegetable broth:** Read the label and make sure it is gluten- and sugar-free. I really like the Pacific Foods Organic brand, which is available in most grocery stores. Or you can make it yourself: See my easy recipe for Poultry, Beef, or Vegetable Stock (page 228).
- **Rice milk:** Choose unflavored (plain) sugar-free rice milk.

Grains

- **Quinoa:** This comes in a variety of types, any of which will do.
- **Brown rice:** Choose the long-cooking brown rice, not the instant variety.
- **Precooked brown rice:** You can find this in the frozen foods section of the grocery store or in the rice section. This is a big time-saver.
- **Steel-cut oats:** Make sure the oats are labeled gluten-free. Some oats are processed on equipment that also processes gluten grains and can be cross-contaminated.

Flours, Seeds, and Sweeteners

- **Coconut flour:** You can find this in the specialty section of most grocery stories, and it is readily available online.
- **Unsweetened cocoa powder:** Check the label to ensure it doesn't contain sugar!
- **Arrowroot powder:** This is an excellent thickener for sauces, puddings, and gravies, working in a manner similar to cornstarch. If you can't find it at the store, it is readily available online.
- **Tapioca powder:** This is a good flour replacement and thickener. You can find this in the specialty flour section at the grocery store and online.
- **Pumpkin seeds:** Choose organic roasted.
- **Chia seed:** Try to find organic.
- **Ground flaxseed:** Try to find organic.
- **Stevia:** Powdered or liquid is fine, although I prefer the latter. I like SweetLeaf Sweet Drops.

A POSITIVE CHANGE

It's true that this is a lot of information to absorb, but these diet and lifestyle changes *will* help you manage your Hashimoto's, and the outcome is totally worth the effort. As you begin to incorporate the changes into your daily life, you should notice positive results. I can attest to this after following the plan that I'm now inviting you to follow. I have more energy, my aches and pains are significantly reduced and often absent, and even my skin looks better than it ever has.

I have designed the recipes to make the dietary changes as easy (and delicious!) as possible for you. Once you have started cooking for yourself, you will see just how easy it can be, and how worthwhile.

7

BREAKFAST

APPLE-CINNAMON OATMEAL

SERVES 4 · PREP TIME: 5 MINUTES · COOK TIME: 5 MINUTES

Oatmeal has a stick-to-your-ribs goodness about it. This version has tasty bits of apples along with fragrant cinnamon and a tiny bit of stevia for sweetness. Made with rice or coconut milk, it's also super creamy and satisfying.

3¼ cups plain unsweetened rice milk

3 drops liquid stevia, or to taste

1 teaspoon ground cinnamon

Pinch sea salt

1 apple, peeled, cored, and cut into small pieces

2 cups steel-cut oats (gluten-free)

1. In a medium pot over medium-high heat, bring the rice milk, stevia, cinnamon, salt, and apple to a boil.

2. Stir in the oats. Cook, stirring frequently, for 3 to 5 minutes, or until the oats are soft.

Ingredient Tip *While you can use any type of apple, a sweet-tart variety, such as a Honeycrisp or Braeburn, has the perfect flavor and texture for this dish. You can also substitute dried apples.*

PER SERVING Calories: 212; Total Fat: 5g; Saturated Fat: <1g; Cholesterol: 0mg; Carbohydrates: 42g; Fiber: 10g; Protein: 6g

SLOW COOKER BREAKFAST RICE

SERVES 4 · PREP TIME: 5 MINUTES · COOK TIME: 8 HOURS

Rice for breakfast? When you combine it with sweet spices and dried fruit, it makes a wonderful start to your day. Best of all, you can put all the ingredients in the slow cooker before you go to bed and wake up to a hot, delicious meal. It's a great way to get ahead of the morning rush.

2 cups brown rice

½ cup raisins

½ cup dried apricots, chopped

2 cups plain unsweetened rice milk

2 cups unsweetened apple juice

1 teaspoon ground cinnamon

⅛ teaspoon ground cloves

1 teaspoon alcohol-free pure vanilla extract

1. Combine all of the ingredients in a slow cooker, stirring well.
2. Put the lid on the slow cooker and set it on low. Cook for 8 hours. Stir before serving.

Variation Tip Add a little bit of protein and crunch by stirring 2 tablespoons raw pumpkin seeds into each bowl of rice just before serving. Pumpkin seeds are an excellent source of zinc, manganese, and magnesium.

PER SERVING Calories: 530; Total Fat: 4g; Saturated Fat: 4g; Cholesterol: 0mg; Carbohydrates: 116g; Fiber: 5g; Protein: 8g

COCONUT FLOUR AND FLAXSEED PORRIDGE

SERVES 2 · PREP TIME: 5 MINUTES · COOK TIME: 3 MINUTES

If you're a Cream of Wheat fan, then you'll like this porridge. The coconut flour, which is a great source of fiber, has a similar texture to that of Cream of Wheat. Flaxseed is an excellent source of potassium, magnesium, and anti-inflammatory omega-3 fatty acids. Adding berries is a great way to boost antioxidants and vitamins.

1½ cups canned lite coconut milk

½ cup coconut flour

2 tablespoons ground flaxseed

4 drops liquid stevia, or to taste

½ cup sliced hulled strawberries

1. In a small saucepan over medium-high heat, combine the coconut milk, coconut flour, ground flaxseed, and stevia and bring to a simmer.
2. Cook, stirring constantly, for 2 to 3 minutes, or until thick.
3. Serve topped with the sliced strawberries.

PER SERVING Calories: 290; Total Fat: 16g; Saturated Fat: 13g; Cholesterol: 0mg; Carbohydrates: 30g; Fiber: 15g; Protein: 10g

COCONUT FLOUR PANCAKES
WITH BERRIES
....

SERVES 4 · PREP TIME: 5 MINUTES · COOK TIME: 10 MINUTES

Just because you're giving up wheat doesn't mean you can't enjoy pancakes. Coconut flour makes a tasty pancake with a flavor that goes perfectly with blueberries. Whether fresh or frozen, blueberries are loaded with antioxidants.

½ cup coconut flour

¼ teaspoon baking powder

Pinch sea salt

2 tablespoons coconut oil, melted

⅔ cup canned lite coconut milk

6 eggs

1 teaspoon alcohol-free pure vanilla extract

3 drops liquid stevia, or to taste

1 cup fresh blueberries

½ cup fresh raspberries

½ cup fresh blackberries

1. In a small bowl, whisk together the coconut flour, baking powder, and salt.

2. In another bowl, whisk together the coconut oil, coconut milk, eggs, vanilla, and stevia.

3. Fold the wet ingredients into the dry ingredients until just combined.

4. Heat a nonstick griddle or sauté pan over medium-high heat.

5. For each pancake, pour ¼ cup of batter onto the griddle.

6. Cook for 3 minutes, or until bubbles form on the surface of the pancakes and the bottom is lightly browned.

7. Using a spatula, flip the pancakes and cook for another 3 minutes, until the bottom is lightly browned.

8. In a small bowl, combine the blueberries, raspberries, and blackberries. Serve the pancakes topped with the mixed berries.

PER SERVING Calories: 270; Total Fat: 18g; Saturated Fat: 12g; Cholesterol: 246mg; Carbohydrates: 17g; Fiber: 7g; Protein: 12g

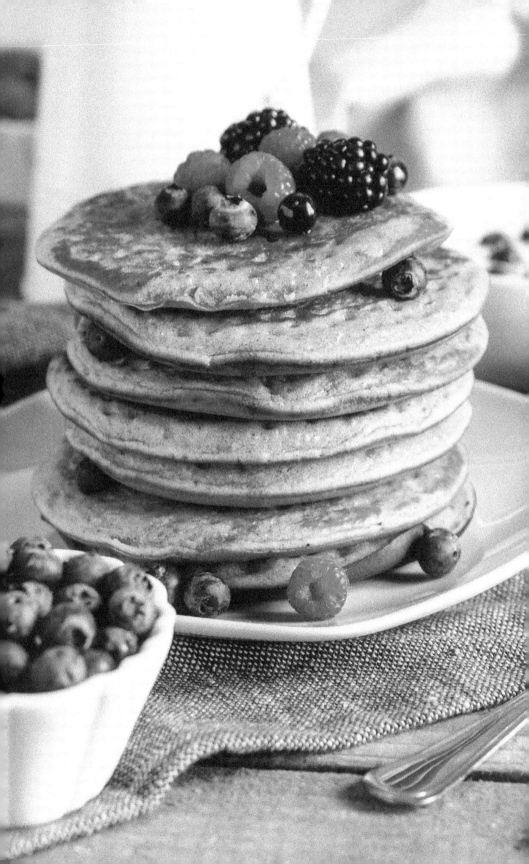

EASY BANANA PANCAKES

....

SERVES 2 · PREP TIME: 5 MINUTES · COOK TIME: 10 MINUTES

This may be the easiest pancake recipe you'll ever see—just three ingredients: bananas, cinnamon, and eggs. The eggs provide protein, while the bananas are high in potassium. Top with fresh berries for a tasty breakfast treat that is super simple to make. I love it when life is this easy!

2 bananas, mashed

4 eggs, beaten

½ teaspoon ground cinnamon

Coconut oil

1 cup fresh raspberries

1. In a small bowl, combine the bananas, eggs, and cinnamon until well mixed.

2. In a nonstick sauté pan or griddle over medium-high heat, melt a small amount of coconut oil and spread it to coat the pan.

3. For each pancake, drop a scant ¼ cup of batter onto the pan.

4. Cook for 3 minutes, or until bubbles form on the surface of the pancakes and the bottom is lightly browned.

5. Using a spatula, flip the pancakes and cook for another 3 minutes, until the bottom is lightly browned.

6. Serve topped with raspberries.

Variation Tip *To make a chocolate banana pancake, stir in 1 tablespoon unsweetened cocoa powder and 4 drops liquid stevia in step 1.*

PER SERVING Calories: 264; Total Fat: 10g; Saturated Fat: 3g; Cholesterol: 327mg; Carbohydrates: 35g; Fiber: 7g; Protein: 13g

PUMPKIN WAFFLES

SERVES 4 · PREP TIME: 5 MINUTES · COOK TIME: 10 MINUTES

In the fall, it seems like people go crazy for pumpkin. It's loaded with nutrients that are great for people with Hashimoto's, including antioxidants, vitamin A, and magnesium. Plus, it tastes so good, particularly when combined with traditional pumpkin pie spices. Who wouldn't want something that tastes like pumpkin pie for breakfast? Top with a dab of Apple Butter (page 225) and dig in. Yum!

1 cup canned pure pumpkin purée (unsweetened)

6 eggs, beaten

½ cup plain unsweetened rice milk

½ teaspoon alcohol-free pure vanilla extract

4 drops liquid stevia, or to taste

1¾ cups tapioca flour

½ cup coconut flour

⅛ teaspoon baking powder

½ teaspoon ground cinnamon

⅛ teaspoon ground nutmeg

⅛ teaspoon ground cloves

Coconut oil

1. In a medium bowl, whisk together the pumpkin purée, eggs, rice milk, vanilla, and stevia.

2. In another bowl, whisk together the tapioca flour, coconut flour, baking powder, cinnamon, nutmeg, and cloves.

3. Carefully fold the wet ingredients into the dry ingredients until just combined.

4. Heat a nonstick waffle iron to medium-high. Lightly grease with coconut oil.

5. For each waffle, pour about ¼ cup of batter into the waffle iron and cook until done, about 4 minutes.

Cooking Tip *If you don't have a waffle iron, you can make these into pancakes instead. For each pancake, drop ¼ cup of batter onto a greased nonstick griddle or sauté pan and cook over medium-high heat for 3 to 4 minutes per side.*

PER SERVING Calories: 262; Total Fat: 9g; Saturated Fat: 4g; Cholesterol: 246mg; Carbohydrates: 34g; Fiber: 6g; Protein: 11g

BAKED AVOCADO WITH SMOKED SALMON AND EGGS

SERVES 2 · PREP TIME: 5 MINUTES · COOK TIME: 20 MINUTES

This simple recipe is the perfect way to start your day. An avocado is halved, hollowed out a bit, lined with smoked salmon, topped with cracked eggs and baked to perfection. Finished with a sprinkling of chopped herbs, and you've got a creamy, decadent-tasting breakfast in no time. If you can find them, choose farm-fresh, free-range eggs, although grocery store eggs will work, as well.

1 avocado, halved and pitted

2 ounces thinly flaked smoked salmon

2 eggs

¼ teaspoon sea salt

¼ teaspoon freshly ground black pepper

1 tablespoon chopped fresh chives

1. Preheat the oven to 425°F.

2. Using a spoon, scoop out just enough avocado flesh to make a hollow big enough to fit one cracked egg and some salmon. Reserve the scooped flesh for another use.

3. Put each avocado half cut-side up in the well of a muffin pan to prevent them from tipping over. Line the hollow of each avocado with an even amount of the salmon.

4. Carefully crack one egg over the top of the salmon in each avocado half.

5. Sprinkle evenly with the salt and pepper.

6. Bake in the preheated oven until the eggs are set, 15 to 20 minutes.

7. Sprinkle with the chives before serving.

Variation Tip You can replace the salmon with thinly sliced ham, crab, or crumbled bacon bits, if you wish.

PER SERVING Calories: 302; Total Fat: 25g; Saturated Fat: 6g; Cholesterol: 170mg; Carbohydrates: 9g; Fiber: 7g; Protein: 13g

MUSHROOM FRITTATA

....

SERVES 4 · PREP TIME: 10 MINUTES · COOK TIME: 10 MINUTES

Earthy, meaty mushrooms are an excellent source of copper and selenium. When combined with the protein in eggs, you'll have a go-to breakfast that gets you moving in the morning. You can use any type of mushrooms in this recipe. I'm a huge fan of shiitake mushrooms or, when they're in season, chanterelles.

2 tablespoons extra-virgin olive oil

8 ounces cremini mushrooms, chopped

½ teaspoon sea salt

⅛ teaspoon freshly ground
  black pepper

½ teaspoon dried thyme

8 eggs

2 tablespoons chopped fresh chives

1. Preheat the oven broiler to high.
2. In a large ovenproof sauté pan over medium-high heat, heat the olive oil until it shimmers.
3. Add the mushrooms, salt, pepper, and thyme. Cook, stirring occasionally, for 5 minutes, or until the mushrooms are well browned.
4. In a small bowl, whisk together the eggs until well beaten.
5. Pour the eggs over the mushrooms. Cook without stirring until the eggs solidify around the edges.
6. Using a rubber spatula, carefully pull the eggs away from the edges of the pan and tilt the pan, allowing any uncooked eggs to run into the gaps. Cook for a few more minutes.
7. Place the pan under the broiler. Cook for 1 to 2 minutes, or until the top of the frittata is browned.
8. Cut into wedges and serve, sprinkled with the chives.

Variation Tip Replace the mushrooms with veggies like chopped zucchini or sautéed spinach. The spinach will take only 1 or 2 minutes to cook.

PER SERVING Calories: 199; Total Fat: 16g; Saturated Fat: 4g; Cholesterol: 327mg; Carbohydrates: 3g; Fiber: <1g; Protein: 13g

EASY EGG, SAUSAGE, AND SWEET POTATO CASSEROLE

SERVES 4 · PREP TIME: 10 MINUTES · COOK TIME: 30 MINUTES

Egg breakfast casseroles keep really well in the refrigerator and reheat in minutes in the microwave. If you double the recipe, use a 9-by-13-inch pan and start checking it after 30 minutes of baking. It's done when it no longer jiggles in the middle.

Coconut oil

8 ounces ground pork

1 teaspoon dried sage

3 garlic cloves, minced

2 cups baby spinach

5 eggs

¼ cup unsweetened plain rice milk

½ teaspoon sea salt

¼ teaspoon freshly ground black pepper

1 sweet potato, peeled and grated

1. Preheat the oven to 400°F. Grease a 9-inch square baking pan with coconut oil.

2. In a medium bowl, combine the ground pork, sage, and garlic until well mixed.

3. In a large nonstick sauté pan over medium-high heat, cook the ground pork mixture, crumbling with a spoon, for 5 minutes or until browned. Add the spinach and cook, stirring occasionally, for 2 minutes. Set aside to cool.

4. In a large bowl, whisk together the eggs, rice milk, salt, and pepper. Fold in the sweet potato and the cooled ground pork mixture.

5. Pour the mixture into the prepared baking pan. Bake in the preheated oven for 20 to 30 minutes, or until the eggs are set.

Variation Tip To make this vegetarian, replace the ground pork with 8 ounces finely chopped mushrooms, browning the mushrooms with the sage and garlic just as you would the pork.

PER SERVING Calories: 201; Total Fat: 8g; Saturated Fat: 2g; Cholesterol: 246mg; Carbohydrates: 9g; Fiber: 1g; Protein: 23g

BACON CUPS WITH BAKED EGGS

SERVES 6 · PREP TIME: 5 MINUTES · COOK TIME: 20 MINUTES

If there were an adorable breakfast contest, this darn-cute-and-really-tasty recipe would win. Not only that, but if you're watching your carbs or eating Paleo, this is the ideal breakfast for you. And it hardly takes any work at all. This recipe also scales well. Whether you've got a 6-cup or 12-cup muffin tin—or a whole pile of muffin tins and want to feed a crowd of 24—this recipe adapts.

12 thin bacon slices

12 eggs

Sea salt

Freshly ground black pepper

1 tablespoon chopped fresh chives

1. Preheat the oven to 350°F.

2. Wrap a slice of bacon around the inside of each muffin cup, leaving the bottom of the tin bacon-free.

3. Carefully crack an egg into each muffin cup.

4. Sprinkle with salt and pepper.

5. Bake in the preheated oven for 20 minutes, or until the bacon is crisp and the eggs are set.

6. Sprinkle with the chopped chives.

Variation Tip *For a lighter dish, use slices of pancetta, Canadian bacon, or prosciutto.*

PER SERVING Calories: 266; Total Fat: 17g; Saturated Fat: 6g; Cholesterol: 357mg; Carbohydrates: >1g; Fiber: 0g; Protein: 25g

8

SMOOTHIES AND SNACKS

PUMPKIN PIE SMOOTHIE

SERVES 2 · PREP TIME: 5 MINUTES · COOK TIME: NONE

If you love pumpkin pie, then you'll enjoy this low-carb, Paleo, vegan smoothie. Classic pumpkin spice flavors are blended with sweet earthy pumpkin purée. You can use either coconut milk or rice milk in this smoothie. Taste as you blend to determine just how much stevia you need for your desired level of sweetness.

2 cups canned lite coconut milk

1½ cups very cold canned pure unsweetened pumpkin purée

½ teaspoon alcohol-free pure vanilla extract

4 drops liquid stevia, or to taste

¼ teaspoon ground cinnamon

⅛ teaspoon ground nutmeg

⅛ teaspoon ground cloves

⅛ teaspoon ground ginger

1. Combine all of the ingredients in a blender.
2. Blend on high speed for 30 seconds, or until smooth.

Ingredient Tip The trick to this smoothie is blending very cold ingredients. Freeze the pumpkin purée in an ice-cube tray and use the cubes in the smoothie.

PER SERVING Calories: 203; Total Fat: 13g; Saturated Fat: 12g; Cholesterol: 0mg; Carbohydrates: 24g; Fiber: 6g; Protein: 5g

SIMPLE GREEN SMOOTHIE

SERVES 2 · PREP TIME: 5 MINUTES · COOK TIME: NONE

Get a healthy dose of your greens in this vegan Paleo smoothie. It is great for breakfast or as a tasty high-energy snack in the afternoon. Adding a little fruit helps mellow the vegetal taste of the greens, while ginger adds a bit of zip.

1 cup canned lite coconut milk

1 cup unsweetened apple juice

2 cups baby spinach

½ avocado

2 cups honeydew melon chunks

½ teaspoon grated peeled fresh ginger

4 drops liquid stevia, or to taste

4 ice cubes

1. Combine all of the ingredients in a blender.
2. Blend on high speed for 30 seconds, or until smooth.

Cooking Tip *If your blender doesn't chop up raw greens well, you can replace the fresh baby spinach with frozen cooked spinach, which will blend better and make your smoothie colder.*

PER SERVING Calories: 298; Total Fat: 16g; Saturated Fat: 8g; Cholesterol: 0mg; Carbohydrates: 40g; Fiber: 6g; Protein: 4g

GINGER-PEACH SMOOTHIE

....

SERVES 2 · PREP TIME: 5 MINUTES · COOK TIME: NONE

Frozen peaches thicken and add a lovely body to this smoothie, while fragrant ginger adds just the right amount of warm spice. (If you like, you can also use frozen nectarines instead of peaches.) The coconut milk provides a nice, creamy base and contains enough fat to keep you feeling satisfied for hours.

1 (14-ounce) can lite coconut milk

2 cups frozen peaches, cubed

1 tablespoon freshly grated peeled ginger

2 drops liquid stevia, or to taste

1. Combine all of the ingredients in a blender.
2. Blend on high speed for 1 minute or until smooth.

Variation Tip *You can use any frozen cubed fruits in this smoothie, such as mango or papaya. To make a Banana Ginger Peach Smoothie, add 1 frozen banana along with ½ cup water.*

PER SERVING Calories: 532; Total Fat: 48g; Saturated Fat: 42g; Cholesterol: 0mg; Carbohydrates: 30g; Fiber: 7g; Protein: 6g

PIÑA COLADA SMOOTHIE

....

SERVES 2 · PREP TIME: 5 MINUTES · COOK TIME: NONE

If you're ready for a tropical break from your day, then you'll love this Paleo piña colada smoothie. It tastes like an afternoon on a beach in Hawaii. Make it whenever you need a mid-winter pick-me-up, or whenever you want something sweet, delicious, and healthy. Don't forget the umbrella for your drink!

2 cups canned coconut milk

2 cups unsweetened
  pineapple chunks

4 drops liquid stevia, or to taste

¼ teaspoon ground nutmeg

½ teaspoon rum extract (optional)

1. Combine all of the ingredients in a blender.

2. Blend on high speed for 30 seconds, or until smooth.

Ingredient Tip *For a nice cold, thick smoothie, freeze the pineapple chunks before adding them to the smoothie. To reduce fat and calories, use lite coconut milk—it won't taste quite as coconutty but will still be delicious.*

PER SERVING Calories: 635; Total Fat: 56g; Saturated Fat: 51g; Cholesterol: 0mg; Carbohydrates: 35g; Fiber: 8g; Protein: 6g

COCONUT GELATIN

SERVES 4 · PREP TIME: 5 MINUTES, PLUS 10 MINUTES TO SIT
COOK TIME: 5 MINUTES, PLUS 2 HOURS TO CHILL

If you've ever been to a luau, then you may be familiar with what I think is the tastiest dish there—coconut gelatin. I'm an admitted coconut fan, and I fell in love with this when I visited my sister in Kauai. Because gelatin is high in protein, I think it makes a pretty ideal low-carb, Paleo snack.

2 cups canned lite coconut milk

8 drops liquid stevia, or to taste

Pinch sea salt

2 tablespoons gelatin

1. In a small saucepan, combine the coconut milk, stevia, and salt.
2. Sprinkle the gelatin over the top of the liquid, spreading it evenly.
3. Let the gelatin sit (bloom) for 10 minutes.
4. Move the saucepan to the stove and, over medium-low heat, gradually bring the mixture to a simmer, stirring constantly.
5. Remove from the heat. Pour into a serving bowl or individual ramekins and refrigerate until the gelatin sets, about 2 hours.

Ingredient Tip My favorite gelatin comes from pastured, organic cattle. It's the Great Lakes unflavored gelatin in the red can. You can find it online.

PER SERVING Calories: 79; Total Fat: 6g; Saturated Fat: 6g; Cholesterol: 0mg; Carbohydrates: 5g; Fiber: 0g; Protein: 5g

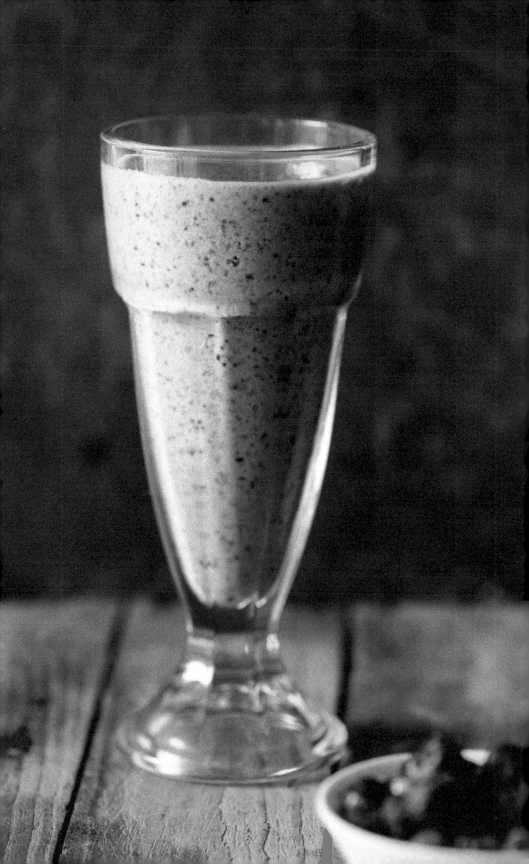

MIXED BERRY-CHIA SMOOTHIE

SERVES 2 · PREP TIME: 5 MINUTES, PLUS 10 MINUTES TO SIT · COOK TIME: NONE

Chia is kind of a cool seed: When it soaks in liquid it turns gelatinous. This makes for a thick smoothie that's high in healthy omega-3 fatty acids and packed with powerful antioxidants. Coconut milk is great if you're opting for a Paleo diet, but if you'd like lower calories and fat, rice milk works just as well.

2 cups canned lite coconut milk

2 tablespoons chia seeds

½ teaspoon alcohol-free pure
  vanilla extract

4 drops liquid stevia, or to taste

2 cups frozen mixed berries

1. In a glass measuring cup, combine the coconut milk and chia seeds. Set aside for 10 minutes.

2. In a blender, combine the milk/chia mixture, vanilla, stevia, and mixed berries.

3. Blend on high speed for 30 seconds, or until smooth.

Variation Tip *For a tropical-treat smoothie, use frozen mango chunks in place of the mixed berries.*

PER SERVING Calories: 374; Total Fat: 22g; Saturated Fat: 13g; Cholesterol: 0mg; Carbohydrates: 41g; Fiber: 15g; Protein: 10g

AVOCADO-GARLIC DEVILED EGGS

SERVES 8 · PREP TIME: 5 MINUTES · COOK TIME: NONE

You can hard-boil the eggs yourself (see the tip below), or you can buy precooked hard-boiled eggs and save yourself time and the hassle of peeling freshly boiled eggs. Either way, these tasty eggs are the perfect snack. They will keep, tightly sealed, in the refrigerator for up to three days.

8 hard-boiled eggs

½ soft avocado, peeled, pitted, and cubed

2 tablespoons Easy Mayonnaise (page 235)

1 tablespoon apple cider vinegar

1 scallion, finely chopped

1 garlic clove, minced

⅛ teaspoon ground turmeric

1. Halve the eggs pole-to-pole (lengthwise). Scoop out the yolks and put them in a small bowl. Set aside the egg whites on a plate, cut-side up.
2. To the egg yolks, add the avocado, mayonnaise, apple cider vinegar, scallion, garlic, and turmeric.
3. Mash the mixture with a fork until smooth.
4. Spoon the mixture into the egg white halves.

Ingredient Tip To hard-boil eggs, put the eggs in a single layer in the bottom of a large pot and cover them with water to an inch above the top of the eggs. Cover with a lid and put the pot on the stove. Over medium-high heat, bring the water to a boil and then immediately remove the pot from the heat. Let the eggs sit in the hot water, covered, for 14 minutes. Remove the eggs from the pot and plunge them into cold water to stop the cooking process.

PER SERVING Calories: 104; Total Fat: 8g; Saturated Fat: 2g; Cholesterol: 165mg; Carbohydrates: 3g; Fiber: >1g; Protein: 6g

JICAMA AND AVOCADO DIP

SERVES 4 · PREP TIME: 5 MINUTES · COOK TIME: NONE

Avocado makes a great nondairy base for creamy dips. Sliced jicama serves as the tasty medium for conveying dip from the bowl to your mouth. Its crunch and mild yet slightly peppery flavor is a perfect counterpoint to the smooth, creamy avocado.

1 avocado, peeled, pitted, and halved

1 cup plain coconut yogurt

Zest of 1 lime

1 tablespoon apple cider vinegar

1 garlic clove, minced

¼ cup chopped fresh cilantro leaves

1 jicama, peeled and sliced

1. In a food process or blender on high speed, purée the avocado, yogurt, lime zest, apple cider vinegar, garlic, and cilantro for 30 seconds, or until smooth.
2. Serve with the sliced jicama.

Ingredient Tip Avocado flesh has a tendency to brown quickly when exposed to air unless acidulated. Traditionally, this is done with citrus juice, but we're using apple cider vinegar instead, which also adds a tangy zip to the dip. To store any leftover dip, put it in a bowl with plastic wrap pressed directly onto the surface of the dip so no air can get to it.

PER SERVING Calories: 192; Total Fat: 12g; Saturated Fat: 4g; Cholesterol: 0mg; Carbohydrates: 22g; Fiber: 14g; Protein: 2g

EASY SWEET POTATO FRIES

SERVES 4 · PREP TIME: 10 MINUTES · COOK TIME: 30 MINUTES

Even though potatoes are a nightshade, you don't have to completely give up French fries. You can make these delightful sweet potato fries instead. While the flavor is slightly sweeter than a potato, I find it infinitely more interesting, and you still get that same delicious, pillowy potato softness of regular fries. Try these with the Avocado Dip on page 153.

2 sweet potatoes, unpeeled and cut into ¼-inch sticks

2 tablespoons coconut oil, melted

1 teaspoon sea salt

¼ teaspoon ground turmeric

1. Preheat the oven to 450°F.
2. In a large bowl, toss the sweet potatoes with the coconut oil, salt, and turmeric.
3. Spread the potatoes in an even layer on a large baking sheet.
4. Bake in the preheated oven, turning twice during cooking, for 25 to 30 minutes, or until the potatoes are crisp and lightly browned on the outside.

Variation Tip This also works well with other root vegetables such as daikon radish or turnips.

PER SERVING Calories: 192; Total Fat: 7g; Saturated Fat: 6g; Cholesterol: 0mg; Carbohydrates: 32g; Fiber: 5g; Protein: 2g

ZUCCHINI HUMMUS

SERVES 4 · PREP TIME: 10 MINUTES · COOK TIME: NONE

I'm a big hummus fan, so I was pretty bummed when I realized that chickpeas were out for me. Then I discovered that you could replace the chickpeas with zucchini for a Paleo, low-carb hummus and still get all the flavors that I totally dig in hummus. This is a simple and fast recipe. Serve it with chopped-up veggies for dipping.

1 zucchini, peeled and chopped	¼ cup tahini
Zest of 1 lemon	2 garlic cloves, minced
2 tablespoons apple cider vinegar	½ teaspoon ground cumin
2 tablespoons extra-virgin olive oil, plus extra for drizzling	¼ teaspoon ground turmeric
	1 teaspoon sea salt

1. Combine all of the ingredients in a food processor or blender.
2. Blend on high speed for 1 minute, or until smooth.
3. Drizzle with additional olive oil before serving.

Variation Tip Tahini is a sesame paste that you can find in most grocery stores. If you don't have tahini, you can replace it with ¼ cup sesame seeds. Put the sesame seeds in the blender and purée them on high speed for a few minutes or until they form a smooth paste. Add the remaining ingredients and purée.

PER SERVING Calories: 163; Total Fat: 15g; Saturated Fat: 2g; Cholesterol: 0mg; Carbohydrates: 6g; Fiber: 2g; Protein: 3g

9

SALADS AND SOUPS

CUCUMBER SALAD WITH GINGER-CILANTRO VINAIGRETTE

SERVES 4 · PREP TIME: 10 MINUTES · COOK TIME: NONE

If you've got a spiralizer, it's fun to make this salad with cucumber noodles, but using a peeler to make ribbons works just as well. The tangy vinaigrette is a great counterpoint to the cool cucumber and sweet carrots. This is an excellent picnic salad or a delicious accompaniment to pork or poultry dishes.

2 cucumbers, peeled

2 carrots, peeled

3 scallions, chopped

¼ cup Ginger-Cilantro Vinaigrette (page 231)

1. Using a vegetable peeler, cut the cucumbers into ribbons by making long peels down the length of the cucumber. Put the slices in a serving bowl. Do the same with the carrots.

2. Add the scallions.

3. Toss with the ginger-cilantro vinaigrette. Serve right away or refrigerate for up to 1 hour to allow the flavors to meld.

Variation Tip This recipe also works well with zucchini or summer squash instead of cucumber.

PER SERVING Calories: 109; Total Fat: 8g; Saturated Fat: 2g; Cholesterol: 0mg; Carbohydrates: 10g; Fiber: 2g; Protein: 1g

COBB SALAD

SERVES 4 · PREP TIME: 15 MINUTES · COOK TIME: NONE

To save time, use precooked rotisserie chicken and precooked hard-boiled eggs to make this salad. Most cobb salads have blue cheese, but we replace the cheese with a refreshing basil vinaigrette.

6 cups romaine lettuce,
  torn into pieces

½ red onion, chopped

4 slices cooked bacon, crumbled

4 hard-boiled eggs, peeled
  and chopped

12 ounces cooked chicken,
  cut into pieces

¼ cup Basil Vinaigrette (page 230)

1. In a large bowl, combine all of the ingredients.
2. Toss to mix.

Variation Tip You can also add chopped tomatoes (once you've discovered whether you're sensitive to nightshades) and raw sunflower seeds to add texture and flavor to the basic salad.

PER SERVING Calories: 481; Total Fat: 23g; Saturated Fat: 6g; Cholesterol: 250mg; Carbohydrates: 5g; Fiber: <1g; Protein: 38g

CREAMY CUCUMBER AND RADISH SALAD

SERVES 4 · PREP TIME: 10 MINUTES · COOK TIME: NONE

This creamy cucumber salad makes a delicious side dish that is both crispy and acidic—a perfect accompaniment to dishes such as Turkey Meatballs (page 194). To cut the cucumber into ribbons, you can use a spiralizer or a vegetable peeler.

2 cucumbers, unpeeled, cut into ribbons

4 radishes, thinly sliced

2 tablespoons Easy Mayonnaise (page 235)

2 tablespoons apple cider vinegar

Zest of 1 lemon

1 garlic clove, minced

1 tablespoon chopped fresh dill

½ teaspoon sea salt

⅛ teaspoon freshly ground black pepper

1. In a large bowl, combine the cucumbers and radishes. Set aside.

2. In a small bowl, whisk together the mayonnaise, apple cider vinegar, lemon zest, garlic, dill, salt, and pepper. Pour over the vegetables and toss to combine.

Variation Tip *This salad is also delicious made with carrot or zucchini ribbons, or a mixture of the two.*

PER SERVING: Calories: 73; Total Fat: 5g; Saturated Fat: 1g; Cholesterol: 3mg; Carbohydrates: 6g; Fiber: 1g; Protein: 1g

LETTUCE CUPS
WITH EGG SALAD

SERVES 4 · PREP TIME: 15 MINUTES · COOK TIME: NONE

Homemade mayonnaise makes this egg salad extra tasty. Adding a little crunch with sunflower seeds and chopped scallions provides textural interest to the salad. This makes a great lunch or snack, and it keeps well, if tightly sealed, for up to four days in the refrigerator.

8 hard-boiled eggs, peeled and chopped

¼ cup raw sunflower seeds, toasted

2 tablespoons chopped fresh tarragon

4 scallions, chopped

½ teaspoon sea salt

¼ teaspoon freshly ground black pepper

¼ cup Easy Mayonnaise (page 235)

4 iceberg lettuce leaves

1. In a large bowl, combine the eggs, sunflower seeds, tarragon, scallions, salt, and pepper. Toss to mix.

2. Stir in the mayonnaise.

3. Serve scooped into the iceberg lettuce cups.

Variation Tip Whisk some freshly grated orange zest into the mayonnaise before adding it to the egg salad. The light citrus flavor marries well with the fresh tarragon.

PER SERVING Calories: 210; Total Fat: 15g; Saturated Fat: 4g; Cholesterol: 331mg; Carbohydrates: 7g; Fiber: <1g; Protein: 12g

FESTIVE FRUIT SALAD

....

SERVES 4 · PREP TIME: 15 MINUTES · COOK TIME: NONE

Fruit salad is a mainstay of the Western diet, and it's easy to see why. Loaded with brightly colored, sweet, juicy fruits, a fruit salad is the perfect light accompaniment for any meal. It also makes a great dessert, or even breakfast dish. Best of all, it doesn't require dressing because the fruit is delicious all by itself. In this recipe, a little bit of black pepper adds bite and contrast to the sweetness of the fruit.

2 cups grapes, halved

2 cups sliced strawberries

2 peaches, pitted and chopped

2 cups chopped honeydew melon

1 apple, cored and chopped

¼ teaspoon freshly ground black pepper (optional)

1. In a large bowl, combine all of the ingredients.

2. Toss to mix. Serve immediately.

Variation Tip *Add 1 teaspoon grated fresh ginger to give this salad a refreshing bite.*

PER SERVING Calories: 128; Total Fat: <1g; Saturated Fat: 0g; Cholesterol: 0mg; Carbohydrates: 32g; Fiber: 4g; Protein: 2g

APPLE-GINGER SLAW

SERVES 4 · PREP TIME: 15 MINUTES · COOK TIME: NONE

*I always thought I hated coleslaw—until I discovered I didn't.
A few years ago, still believing I didn't like coleslaw, I decided I'd
give it one more try using apples and jicama. The result made
me a believer. Give this one a try. It makes a refreshing side dish
or snack.*

2 sweet-tart apples, peeled, cored, and julienned

1 small jicama, peeled and julienned

1 tablespoon grated peeled ginger

3 tablespoons extra-virgin olive oil

1 tablespoon apple cider vinegar

¼ teaspoon sea salt

2 drops liquid stevia, or to taste

1. In a large bowl, toss together the apple and jicama.
2. In a small bowl, whisk together the ginger, olive oil, apple cider vinegar, salt, and stevia.
3. Toss the vinaigrette with the apples and jicama.

Variation Tip *Add 1 teaspoon finely grated orange or lime zest to the vinaigrette to give this salad a citrus zing.*

PER SERVING Calories: 205; Total Fat: 11g; Saturated Fat: 2g; Cholesterol: 0mg; Carbohydrates: 28g; Fiber: 10g; Protein: 2g

AVGOLEMONO SOUP WITH LAMB

SERVES 4 · PREP TIME: 10 MINUTES · COOK TIME: 20 MINUTES

Avgolemono, a Greek egg-and-lemon sauce, has a delicious acidity that combines beautifully with the gamey flavor of ground lamb. This delicious and hearty soup features traditional avgolemono flavors, along with earthy Greek herbs and spices.

2 tablespoons extra-virgin olive oil	6 cups Beef Broth (page 228)
1 pound ground lamb	6 eggs
1 tablespoon dried rosemary	Juice of 3 lemons
1 tablespoon dried oregano	1 teaspoon sea salt
1 onion, chopped	⅛ teaspoon freshly ground black pepper
5 garlic cloves, minced	

1. In a large pot over medium-high heat, heat the olive oil until it shimmers.
2. Add the lamb and cook, breaking it up with the back of a spoon, until browned, about 5 minutes.
3. Stir in the rosemary, oregano, and onion. Cook, stirring occasionally, until the onion is soft, about 3 minutes.
4. Add the garlic and cook, stirring constantly, for 30 seconds.
5. Add the beef broth. Bring the soup to a simmer and simmer for 5 minutes. Turn off the heat.
6. In a small bowl, whisk together the eggs, lemon juice, salt, and pepper.
7. While stirring the soup constantly, pour the lemon mixture into the soup in a very thin stream (the egg should cook into thin strands). Serve immediately.

Variation Tip *If you'd like to add some green to this soup, stir in 2 cups baby spinach in step 7, just after you add the egg and lemon mixture. The residual heat of the soup will wilt the spinach.*

PER SERVING Calories: 457; Total Fat: 25g; Saturated Fat: 7g; Cholesterol: 348mg; Carbohydrates: 8g; Fiber: 2g; Protein: 49g

PUMPKIN SOUP WITH SAGE

SERVES 4 · PREP TIME: 15 MINUTES · COOK TIME: 15 MINUTES

*Using canned pumpkin purée makes this soup a breeze. I love
how the flavor of the sage pairs with the sweet, earthy pumpkin
to make a creamy and satisfying Paleo, vegan, low-carb soup.*

2 tablespoons extra-virgin olive oil

2 shallots, minced

2 garlic cloves, minced

4 cups Vegetable Broth (page 228)

1 (29-ounce) can pure (unsweetened)
   pumpkin purée

1 teaspoon ground sage

Pinch ground nutmeg

¼ cup canned coconut milk

½ teaspoon sea salt

¼ teaspoon freshly ground
   black pepper

1. In a large saucepan over medium-high heat, heat the olive oil
   until it shimmers.

2. Add the shallots and cook, stirring occasionally, for 3 minutes,
   or until soft.

3. Add the garlic and cook, stirring constantly, until fragrant.

4. Add the vegetable broth. Whisk in the pumpkin, sage,
   and nutmeg.

5. Stirring frequently, bring to a simmer (it should take
   about 5 minutes). Simmer for an additional 5 minutes,
   stirring frequently.

6. Stir in the coconut milk, salt, and pepper. Heat through
   and serve hot.

Variation Tip *Replace the sage with an equal amount of ground fennel
seeds, and garnish the soup with a sprinkling of fennel seeds, a dollop of
coconut cream, and a fennel sprig.*

PER SERVING Calories: 224; Total Fat: 13g; Saturated Fat: 5g; Cholesterol: 0mg;
Carbohydrates: 23g; Fiber: 6g; Protein: 8g

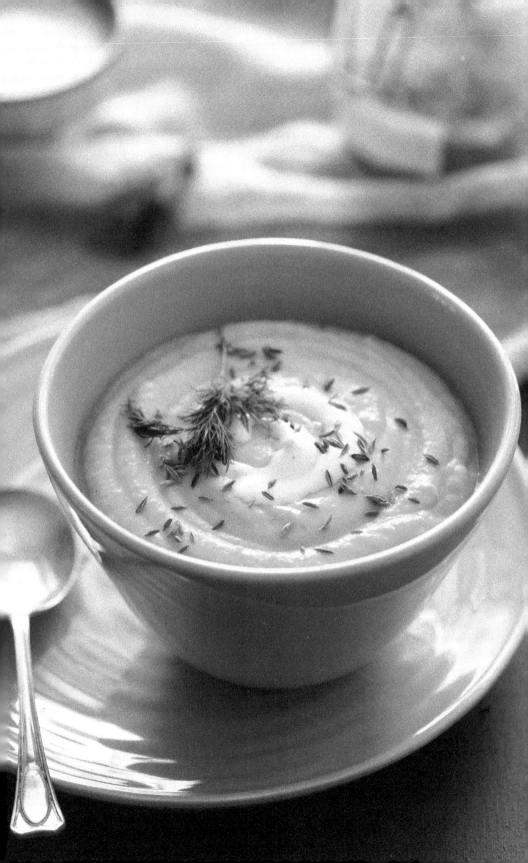

MUSHROOM SOUP

SERVES 4 · PREP TIME: 10 MINUTES, PLUS 2 HOURS TO REST
COOK TIME: 30 MINUTES

Mushrooms are one of my favorite foods in the entire world, and I really love them in soup. They have an earthy flavor and meaty texture that is warm and satisfying. While this soup calls for cremini and porcini mushrooms, you can choose any favorite variety. Shiitake or button mushrooms are excellent, as are any wild mushrooms you can find.

6 cups Chicken Broth (page 228)

4 ounces dried porcini mushrooms

3 tablespoons extra-virgin olive oil

4 ounces pancetta, chopped

2 shallots, minced

1 pound cremini mushrooms, sliced

1 teaspoon dried thyme

1 teaspoon sea salt

¼ teaspoon freshly ground black pepper

1. In a saucepan over medium-high heat, heat the chicken broth until it boils. Remove from the heat. Stir in the porcini mushrooms and set aside for 2 hours.

2. Using a slotted spoon, remove the porcini mushrooms from the broth and roughly chop them. Set aside the mushrooms and broth separately.

3. In a large pot over medium-high heat, heat the olive oil until it shimmers.

4. Add the pancetta and cook, stirring occasionally, for 5 minutes, or until browned.

5. Remove the pancetta with a slotted spoon and set it aside.

6. Add the shallots to the hot oil and cook, stirring occasionally, until soft, about 3 minutes.

7. Add the cremini and reserved porcini mushrooms and cook, stirring occasionally, for 8 minutes, or until well browned.

8. Add the reserved broth, pancetta, thyme, salt, and pepper to the pot, scraping any browned bits from the bottom of the pot with the edge of a spoon.

9. Simmer, stirring occasionally, for 5 minutes.

Ingredient Tip *Mushrooms are like little sponges, so if you wash them with water, they'll soak it up and won't brown easily. Instead, clean the mushrooms using a soft, dry cloth or mushroom brush, wiping away any dirt.*

PER SERVING Calories: 399; Total Fat: 23g; Saturated Fat: 5g; Cholesterol: 31mg; Carbohydrates: 23g; Fiber: 8g; Protein: 21g

COCONUT AND
LEMONGRASS SHRIMP SOUP

SERVES 4 · PREP TIME: 10 MINUTES · COOK TIME: 30 MINUTES

I'm a huge fan of Asian flavor profiles, like the coconut and lemongrass in this soup. You can buy lemongrass paste in a tube in the produce section of your grocery store, and it's a great way to flavor your soup without going to the trouble of chopping up lemongrass yourself.

2 tablespoons coconut oil

1 onion, chopped

4 garlic cloves, minced

4 cups Chicken or Vegetable Broth (page 228)

1 pound shiitake mushrooms, sliced

1 tablespoon lemongrass paste

1 pound shrimp, peeled, deveined, tails removed

1 teaspoon sea salt

¼ teaspoon freshly ground black pepper

1 (14-ounce) can coconut milk

2 tablespoons chopped fresh cilantro leaves (optional)

1. In a large pot over medium-high heat, heat the coconut oil until it shimmers.

2. Add the onion and cook, stirring occasionally, for 5 minutes, or until soft.

3. Add the garlic and cook, stirring constantly, for 30 seconds, or until fragrant.

4. Add the chicken or vegetable broth, shiitake mushrooms, and lemongrass paste. Stir to combine.

5. Bring the mixture to a simmer, stirring occasionally (it should take about 5 minutes). Simmer for an additional 10 minutes.

6. Stir in the shrimp, salt, and pepper. Cook for 5 minutes, or until the shrimp is pink.

7. Stir in the coconut milk and cilantro, if using. Bring to a simmer, stirring constantly (it should take about 2 minutes).

8. Serve immediately.

Variation Tip *To make this dish vegetarian, replace the shrimp with 2 sweet potatoes that have been peeled and cubed. Add the potatoes with the mushrooms in step 4 and simmer for 15 minutes, or until they are soft, before continuing with step 5.*

PER SERVING Calories: 743; Total Fat: 40g; Saturated Fat: 32g; Cholesterol: 347mg; Carbohydrates: 27g; Fiber: 6g; Protein: 71g

GROUND BEEF SOUP WITH CARAMELIZED ONIONS AND CARAWAY

....

SERVES 4 · PREP TIME: 15 MINUTES · COOK TIME: 45 MINUTES

When I discovered that I couldn't eat gluten any longer because of my celiac disease, I knew I was going to miss patty melt sandwiches. I love the way the flavors of caraway, caramelized onions, and mustard mixed so well. Then I came up with this soup, which has those flavors without the gluten. It's a pretty tasty version of the patty melt.

3 tablespoons extra-virgin olive oil

2 onions, thinly sliced

1 pound ground beef

2 garlic cloves, minced

6 cups Beef Broth (page 228)

1 tablespoon mustard powder

1 teaspoon ground caraway

1 teaspoon sea salt

¼ teaspoon freshly ground black pepper

1. In a large pot over medium-high heat, heat the olive oil until it shimmers.

2. Reduce the heat to low. Add the onions. Cook, stirring occasionally, for 30 minutes, or until they are caramelized.

3. Using a slotted spoon, remove the onions from the pot and set aside. Increase the heat to medium-high.

4. Add the ground beef and cook, crumbling with a spoon, for 5 minutes, or until browned.

5. Add the garlic and cook, stirring constantly, for 30 seconds, or until fragrant.

6. Add the beef broth, using the edge of a spoon to scrape any browned bits from the bottom of the pot.

7. Add the mustard powder, caraway, salt, and pepper. Bring to a simmer and cook, stirring occasionally, for 10 minutes.

8. Stir in the reserved onions and serve.

Variation Tip *I really like adding sliced mushrooms to this dish for a little extra texture and flavor. Add 8 ounces sliced mushrooms in step 6. You can also add a little cheesy flavor by sprinkling a few teaspoons of nutritional yeast over the top of the soup when you serve it.*

PER SERVING Calories: 398; Total Fat: 21g; Saturated Fat: 5g; Cholesterol: 101mg; Carbohydrates: 8g; Fiber: 2g; Protein: 43g

10

VEGETARIAN DINNERS

SWEET POTATO, SHIITAKE, AND SPINACH CURRY

SERVES 4 · PREP TIME: 10 MINUTES · COOK TIME: 20 MINUTES

This coconut curry is nutritious and warming, with tender sweet potatoes, hearty shiitake mushrooms, and nutritious spinach. Spinach is a great food to eat when you are iron deficient, and the vitamin C in the spinach and sweet potatoes will help with the absorption of the iron. Serve with steamed brown rice, if you wish.

2 tablespoons coconut oil

3 tablespoons red curry paste

1 onion, chopped

1 pound shiitake mushrooms, sliced

2 sweet potatoes, peeled and cubed

3 cups Vegetable Broth (page 228)

2 cups baby spinach

1 (14-ounce) can coconut milk

1 teaspoon sea salt

1. In a large pot over medium-high heat, heat the coconut oil until it shimmers.

2. Add the red curry paste and the onion. Cook, stirring frequently, for 3 minutes.

3. Add the shiitake mushrooms, sweet potatoes, and vegetable broth. Cook, stirring occasionally, for 15 minutes, or until the potatoes are tender.

4. Add the spinach, coconut milk, and salt. Cook, stirring constantly, for 1 to 2 minutes, or until the spinach wilts and the curry is warmed through.

Variation Tip Replace the sweet potatoes with 3 cups cubed butternut squash for a sweeter version of this curry.

PER SERVING Calories: 613; Total Fat: 36g; Saturated Fat: 28g; Cholesterol: 0mg; Carbohydrates: 69g; Fiber: 12g; Protein: 11g

GARLIC AND SPINACH ZUCCHINI RIBBONS

....

SERVES 4 · PREP TIME: 10 MINUTES, PLUS 15 MINUTES TO DRAIN
COOK TIME: 10 MINUTES

There's no need to miss pasta when zucchini can fill in quite nicely, thank you very much. I'm a huge zucchini-as-noodles fan myself— I make a lot of "pasta" dishes by cutting zucchini into all kinds of shapes. Here, you can use a vegetable peeler to make ribbons, or you can get fancy and spiralize the zucchini into "spaghetti." Either way, it's a solid and tasty dish that's ready quickly.

3 zucchini

1 teaspoon sea salt, plus additional
  for sprinkling

3 tablespoons extra-virgin olive oil

2 tablespoons minced shallot

6 garlic cloves, minced

3 cups baby spinach

¼ cup Vegetable Broth (page 228)

¼ teaspoon freshly ground
  black pepper

2 tablespoons chopped fresh basil

1. Using a vegetable peeler, peel down the length of the zucchini to make ribbons (or use a spiralizer to make noodles).

2. Put the zucchini in a colander placed over the sink or a bowl, sprinkle the zucchini with salt, and let it drain for 15 minutes. This will draw excess water out of the zucchini. Wipe the salt away with paper towels and set the zucchini aside.

3. In a large sauté pan over medium-high heat, heat the olive oil until it shimmers.

4. Add the shallot and cook, stirring occasionally, for 3 minutes, or until soft.

5. Add the garlic and cook, stirring constantly, for 30 seconds, or until fragrant.

6. Add the reserved zucchini and cook, stirring occasionally, for 3 minutes.

7. Add the spinach, vegetable broth, 1 teaspoon of salt, and pepper and cook, stirring occasionally, for 1 to 2 minutes, or until the spinach wilts.

8. Remove from the heat and stir in the fresh basil.

Variation Tip *If you like the taste of Parmesan cheese on your pasta, then sprinkle 1 tablespoon nutritional yeast over the pasta once it is cooked.*

PER SERVING Calories: 132; Total Fat: 11g; Saturated Fat: 2g; Cholesterol: 0mg; Carbohydrates: 8g; Fiber: 2g; Protein: 3g

VEGGIE AND RICE STIR-FRY

SERVES 4 · PREP TIME: 10 MINUTES · COOK TIME: 15 MINUTES

The great thing about stir-fries is that they come together quickly and have endless variations. To save time, use precooked brown rice, which you can find in the freezer and rice sections of the grocery store. You can also cook the rice yourself ahead of time and freeze 1-cup servings in zipper-close bags.

2 tablespoons coconut oil

1 leek, white and light green parts only, sliced

2 large carrots, peeled and sliced

1 pound shiitake mushrooms, sliced

4 eggs, beaten

2 cups cooked brown rice

2 tablespoons gluten-free soy sauce or tamari

1 teaspoon grated peeled ginger

2 garlic cloves, minced

1. In a large sauté pan over medium-high heat, heat the coconut oil until it shimmers.

2. Add the leek, carrots, and mushrooms and cook, stirring frequently, for 5 minutes, or until the vegetables begin to brown.

3. Add the eggs and cook, stirring constantly, for 3 minutes, or until the egg solidifies.

4. Add the brown rice.

5. In a small bowl, whisk together the soy sauce, ginger, and garlic. Add to the rice mixture. Cook, stirring frequently, for 4 minutes, or until the rice is warmed through.

Variation Tip *To make this vegan, omit the egg.*

PER SERVING Calories: 369; Total Fat: 13g; Saturated Fat: 7g; Cholesterol: 164mg; Carbohydrates: 57g; Fiber: 6g; Protein: 13g

MINTED QUINOA AND VEGETABLES

....

SERVES 4 · PREP TIME: 10 MINUTES · COOK TIME: 25 MINUTES

Quinoa has a nutty taste. It's also high in protein, so it makes a filling and satisfying meal. This vegan quinoa dish doesn't have a lot of active time, so it comes together quickly. You can add any vegetables that appeal to you, or keep it simple with the ingredients listed below. The dish also freezes well, so it's a particularly good choice for making in big batches for lunches and dinners on the go.

1 cup quinoa, rinsed and drained (see Ingredient Tip)

2 cups Vegetable Broth (page 228)

2 tablespoons coconut oil

4 scallions, chopped

1 zucchini, chopped

8 ounces shiitake mushrooms, chopped

1 teaspoon sea salt

¼ teaspoon freshly ground black pepper

2 tablespoons chopped fresh mint

1. In a large saucepan over medium-high heat, bring the quinoa and vegetable broth to a boil. Reduce the heat to low, cover, and simmer for 15 minutes. Fluff with a fork. Set aside.

2. In a large sauté pan over medium-high heat, heat the coconut oil until it shimmers. Add the scallions, zucchini, and mushrooms and cook, stirring occasionally, for 7 minutes, or until the vegetables begin to brown.

3. Stir in the quinoa, salt, and pepper. Remove from the heat and stir in the mint.

Ingredient Tip Quinoa can be bitter if not rinsed properly. Put the quinoa in a fine-mesh strainer and run it under cold water, agitating it with your hands to rinse away bitter residues.

PER SERVING Calories: 201; Total Fat: 9g; Saturated Fat: 6g; Cholesterol: 0mg; Carbohydrates: 25g; Fiber: 4g; Protein: 7g

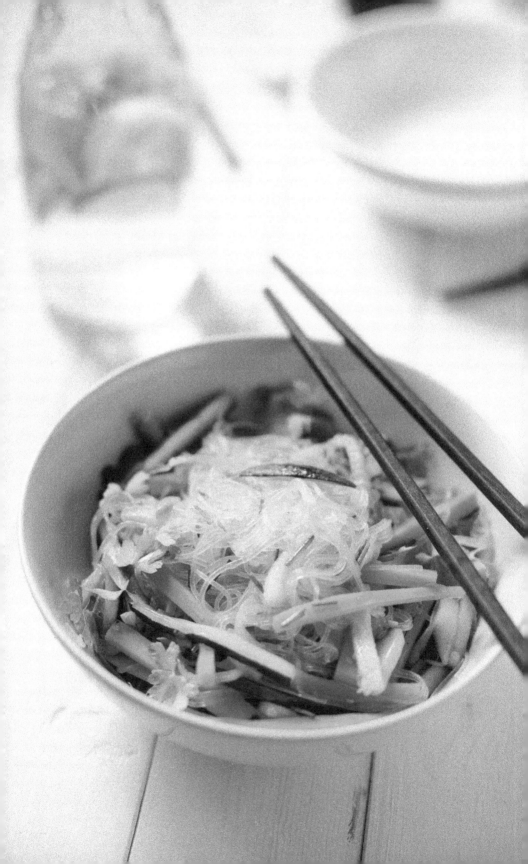

RICE NOODLES AND VEGETABLE STIR-FRY

SERVES 4 · PREP TIME: 10 MINUTES · COOK TIME: 10 MINUTES

Rice noodles, which cook quickly when submerged in boiling-hot water, make this dish a cinch to prepare. The simple marinade adds lots of flavor to the veggies and noodles, while the vegetables are an excellent source of nutrients. Feel free to substitute any veggies you like, or even add shiitake mushrooms, to make this tasty stir-fry your own.

2 tablespoons coconut oil

2 scallions, thinly sliced

1 zucchini, julienned

1 yellow squash, julienned

2 carrots, peeled and julienned

1 garlic clove, minced

1 tablespoon grated peeled ginger

2 tablespoons rice vinegar

½ teaspoon expeller-pressed sesame oil

Zest of 1 lime

1 teaspoon arrowroot powder

2 cups dried rice noodles, cooked according to package directions and drained

3 tablespoons chopped fresh cilantro leaves

1. In a large sauté pan over medium-high heat, heat the coconut oil until it shimmers.

2. Add the scallions, zucchini, yellow squash, and carrots and cook, stirring occasionally, just until the vegetables are crisp-tender, 3 to 4 minutes.

3. Add the garlic and ginger and cook, stirring constantly, for 1 minute, until fragrant.

4. In a small bowl, whisk together the rice vinegar, sesame oil, lime juice, and arrowroot powder. Add to the pan along with the drained rice noodles and cook, stirring constantly, for 1 minute or until heated through.

5. Stir in the cilantro and serve immediately.

PER SERVING Calories: 204; Total Fat: 8g; Saturated Fat: 6g; Cholesterol: 0mg; Carbohydrates: 32g; Fiber: 3g; Protein: 3g

STUFFED ZUCCHINI BOATS

This simple quinoa and mushroom stuffing is fragrant with herbs, making it a delicious filling for hollowed-out zucchini boats. Most of the cooking time is downtime, so you can quickly get your zucchini boats in the oven and settle down with your feet up until it's time to eat. For extra ease, cook up a large batch of quinoa ahead of time and freeze 1-cup portions in zipper-close bags.

½ cup quinoa, rinsed and drained (see Ingredient Tip on page 177)

1 cup Vegetable Broth (page 228)

4 medium zucchini

2 tablespoons extra-virgin olive oil

2 tablespoons minced shallot

8 ounces cremini mushrooms, finely chopped

1 teaspoon dried thyme

1 teaspoon sea salt

¼ teaspoon freshly ground black pepper

4 garlic cloves, minced

1. In a large saucepan over medium-high heat, bring the quinoa and vegetable broth to a boil. Reduce the heat to low, cover, and simmer for 15 minutes. Fluff with a fork. Set aside.

2. Preheat the oven to 350°F.

3. For each zucchini, cut off a lengthwise strip to form the top of the boat. Scoop out some of the flesh to make room for the stuffing. Finely chop all of the trimmings and set aside.

4. Put the zucchini boats on a baking sheet. It might be necessary to shave a sliver of skin off the bottom of the boats so that they sit flat.

5. In a large sauté pan over medium-high heat, heat the olive oil until it shimmers. Add the shallot, mushrooms, chopped zucchini trimmings, thyme, salt, and pepper. Cook, stirring occasionally, for 7 minutes, or until the vegetables are well browned.

6. Add the garlic and cook, stirring constantly, for 30 seconds, or until fragrant.

7. Spoon the stuffing evenly into the zucchini boats. Cover with aluminum foil and bake in the preheated oven for 45 minutes, or until the zucchini is soft.

Variation Tip *Replace the zucchini with pattypan squash, but create a hollow for the stuffing by trimming and scooping from the top. Bake as directed.*

PER SERVING Calories: 204; Total Fat: 9g; Saturated Fat: 1g; Cholesterol: 0mg; Carbohydrates: 25g; Fiber: 4g; Protein: 8g

ASPARAGUS QUICHE

SERVES 4 · PREP TIME: 10 MINUTES · COOK TIME: 45 MINUTES

A crustless quiche is a very easy and quick dish to make. This version has tasty asparagus, which is an excellent source of vitamin K, folate, copper, selenium, and B vitamins, so it's great for people with Hashimoto's. It also keeps well either in the fridge or freezer for a great make-it-and-take-it meal.

2 tablespoons extra-virgin olive oil

½ onion, chopped

1 bunch asparagus, trimmed and chopped (see Ingredient Tip)

2 garlic cloves, minced

8 eggs, beaten

¼ cup plain unsweetened rice milk

½ teaspoon sea salt

¼ teaspoon freshly ground black pepper

1. Preheat the oven to 350°F.

2. In a large sauté pan over medium-high heat, heat the olive oil until it shimmers. Add the onion and asparagus and cook, stirring occasionally, for 7 minutes, or until the asparagus is soft.

3. Add the garlic and cook, stirring constantly, for 30 seconds, or until fragrant. Set aside to cool slightly.

4. In a bowl, mix together the eggs, rice milk, salt, and pepper.

5. Combine the vegetable mixture with the egg mixture, and pour into a 9-inch square baking pan.

6. Bake in the preheated oven for 45 minutes, or until the eggs are set.

Ingredient Tip *To trim asparagus, hold each end of a spear between the thumb and forefinger of each hand. Bend gently until the asparagus breaks. Discard the tough end and keep the tender end.*

PER SERVING Calories: 222; Total Fat: 16g; Saturated Fat: 4g; Cholesterol: 327mg; Carbohydrates: 8g; Fiber: 3g; Protein: 14g

PESTO ZOODLES

SERVES 4 · PREP TIME: 10 MINUTES, PLUS 15 MINUTES TO DRAIN
COOK TIME: 10 MINUTES

A julienne peeler or spiralizer is best for making these noodles, although you can do it by hand. To make the zoodles by hand, use a vegetable peeler to cut long strips of zucchini, and then use a paring knife to cut the strips into spaghetti-sized noodles. The pesto uses pumpkin seeds in place of pine nuts. Pumpkin seeds are an excellent source of zinc, iron, and magnesium.

3 medium zucchini, cut into noodles

¾ teaspoon salt, plus additional for sprinkling

¼ cup plus 2 tablespoons extra-virgin olive oil, divided

1½ cups raw pumpkin seeds

3 garlic cloves, minced

1 cup loosely packed fresh basil leaves

¼ cup nutritional yeast

1. Put the zucchini in a colander placed over the sink or a bowl, sprinkle the zucchini with salt, and let drain for 15 minutes. This will draw excess water out of the zucchini. Wipe the salt away with paper towels and set the zucchini aside.

2. In a food processor or blender, combine ¼ cup of olive oil, pumpkin seeds, garlic, basil, and nutritional yeast. Blend on high speed for 1 minute, or until the seeds and basil are chopped. Set aside.

3. In a large sauté pan over medium-high heat, heat the remaining 2 tablespoons of olive oil until it shimmers. Add the zucchini noodles and cook, stirring occasionally, for 3 minutes, or until the noodles are soft.

4. Toss the noodles with the pesto and serve.

Variation Tip To make spinach pesto, replace the pumpkin seeds with an equal amount of raw sunflower seeds, and replace half of the basil with baby spinach.

PER SERVING Calories: 512; Total Fat: 44g; Saturated Fat: 7g; Cholesterol: 0mg; Carbohydrates: 20g; Fiber: 6g; Protein: 19g

SWEET POTATO HASH BROWNS WITH SAUTÉED MUSHROOMS

SERVES 4 · PREP TIME: 10 MINUTES · COOK TIME: 20 MINUTES

Top these crispy, flavorful sweet potato cakes with earthy mushrooms and a hint of thyme. Mushrooms are a great source of several of the nutrients people with Hashimoto's need, such as copper and selenium, so finding ways to add them to your diet helps ensure you get the nutrients you need. If you'd like a little extra protein, top this with a fried egg.

6 tablespoons extra-virgin olive oil, divided

2 sweet potatoes, peeled and grated

1 teaspoon sea salt, divided

½ teaspoon freshly ground black pepper, divided

8 ounces cremini mushrooms, chopped

½ teaspoon dried thyme

2 garlic cloves, minced

1. Preheat the oven to 200°F.

2. In a large sauté pan over medium-high heat, heat 3 tablespoons of olive oil until it shimmers.

3. Add the sweet potatoes in a single layer, and sprinkle them with ½ teaspoon of salt and ¼ teaspoon of pepper. Cook without moving the potatoes for 5 minutes, or until browned.

4. With a spatula, flip the potatoes and cook the second side for 5 minutes, or until browned. Remove from the pan and set aside on an ovenproof plate in the preheated oven to keep warm.

5. Return the pan to the heat. Add the remaining 3 tablespoons of olive oil and heat until it shimmers.

6. Add the mushrooms, thyme, remaining ½ teaspoon of salt, and remaining ¼ teaspoon of pepper. Cook, stirring very occasionally, for 7 minutes, or until the mushrooms are browned.

7. Add the garlic and cook, stirring constantly, for 30 seconds, or until fragrant.

8. Serve the hash browns topped with the mushrooms.

Variation Tip *Not a fan of sweet potatoes? No worries! Replace the sweet potatoes with 2 cups grated zucchini.*

PER SERVING Calories: 331; Total Fat: 21g; Saturated Fat: 3g; Cholesterol: 0mg; Carbohydrates: 35g; Fiber: 5g; Protein: 3g

SAUTÉED SPINACH
WITH FRIED EGGS

SERVES 2 · PREP TIME: 5 MINUTES · COOK TIME: 10 MINUTES

This is a really simple, yet very satisfying, meal. Sautéed greens are high in iron, and the fried egg provides satisfying protein. With garlic and a little bit of orange zest in the spinach, it's tangy and delicious as a fast and filling weeknight meal. Fry the egg any way you like—I'm a sucker for over easy with a runny yolk, but if your preference is less runny, just adjust the cooking time (see the Cooking Tip).

2 tablespoons extra-virgin olive oil

6 cups baby spinach

½ teaspoon sea salt, plus a pinch

¼ teaspoon freshly ground
  black pepper, plus a pinch

4 garlic cloves, minced

Zest of 1 orange

4 eggs

1. In a large, nonstick sauté pan over medium-high heat, heat the olive oil until it shimmers.

2. Add the spinach, ½ teaspoon of salt, and ¼ teaspoon of pepper and cook, stirring constantly, for 2 minutes, or until the spinach wilts.

3. Add the garlic and orange zest and cook, stirring constantly, for 30 seconds. Spoon the spinach onto two plates.

4. Reduce the heat to medium. Crack four eggs into the pan. Sprinkle the eggs with a pinch each of salt and pepper. Without moving the eggs, cook for 3 minutes, or until the whites are solid.

5. Using a spatula, carefully flip the eggs. Turn the heat off under the pan and, for over-easy style, leave the eggs in the pan for 60 seconds.

6. Using a spatula, carefully place two eggs on top of each portion of spinach.

Cooking Tip *For over-medium eggs, leave the turned eggs in the hot pan for 2 minutes. For over-hard eggs, leave the turned eggs in the hot pan for 3 minutes.*

PER SERVING Calories: 275; Total Fat: 23g; Saturated Fat: 5g; Cholesterol: 327mg; Carbohydrates: 6g; Fiber: 2g; Protein: 14g

11

POULTRY AND MEAT DINNERS

SLOW COOKER CHICKEN AND MUSHROOM STEW

....

SERVES 4 · PREP TIME: 10 MINUTES · COOK TIME: 8 HOURS

Use skin-on chicken thighs in this recipe for an appealing mouthfeel and savory meatiness. For slow cooking, thighs work better than breasts; the fat in thighs keeps the meat moist while breasts tend to dry out. If you don't like chicken skin, remove it before serving. If you wish, serve this dish spooned over cooked brown rice.

8 bone-in, skin-on chicken thighs

1 onion, chopped

1 pound cremini mushrooms, quartered

4 carrots, peeled and chopped

1 fennel bulb, chopped

2 cups Chicken Broth (page 228)

1 teaspoon garlic powder

1 teaspoon dried thyme

1 teaspoon sea salt

¼ teaspoon freshly ground black pepper

1. Put all of the ingredients in a slow cooker and stir to combine.

2. Turn the slow cooker on low. Cover and cook for 8 hours.

Ingredient Tip Fennel is a versatile vegetable. While this recipe calls for only the bulb (the bottom part), you can also cut up the stalks and use them like celery, or mince the fronds as a seasoning. If you like, garnish this dish with chopped fennel fronds for a hit of fresh flavor.

PER SERVING Calories: 648; Total Fat: 22g; Saturated Fat: 6g; Cholesterol: 260mg; Carbohydrates: 18g; Fiber: 5g; Protein: 89g

EASY ROAST CHICKEN WITH ROOT VEGETABLES

....

SERVES 4 · PREP TIME: 10 MINUTES · COOK TIME: 50 MINUTES

Roasting this bird takes awhile, so you'll have plenty of time to relax before dinner as it cooks. Aside from 10 minutes of prep time in the beginning, this is a low-effort meal that looks like you made a fuss.

4 large carrots, peeled and chopped

1 sweet potato, peeled and cut into cubes

6 shallots, peeled and quartered

4 tablespoons extra-virgin olive oil, divided

2½ teaspoons sea salt, divided

½ teaspoon freshly ground black pepper, divided

2 teaspoons dried rosemary

1 teaspoon dried thyme

3 garlic cloves, minced

1 whole roaster chicken (3½- to 5-pound)

1. Preheat the oven to 375°F.

2. In an ovenproof Dutch oven, toss the carrots, sweet potato, and shallots with 2 tablespoons of olive oil, ½ teaspoon of salt, and ¼ teaspoon of pepper.

3. In a small bowl, combine the remaining 2 tablespoons of olive oil, the remaining 2 teaspoons of salt, the remaining ¼ teaspoon of pepper, and the rosemary, thyme, and garlic. Rub the olive oil mixture on the outside of the chicken and put the chicken in the Dutch oven, breast-side up, arranging the vegetables around the chicken.

4. Cover the Dutch oven and bake in the preheated oven for 40 minutes. Uncover and increase the oven temperature to 425°F. Bake for a further 10 minutes, or until the temperature in the meaty part of the chicken leg reaches 180°F.

5. Let the chicken rest for 10 minutes before carving.

PER SERVING Calories: 322; Total Fat: 16g; Saturated Fat: 3g; Cholesterol: 55mg; Carbohydrates: 22g; Fiber: 3g; Protein: 23g

TURKEY BURGERS, PROTEIN STYLE

SERVES 4 · PREP TIME: 5 MINUTES · COOK TIME: 30 MINUTES

Paleo dieters know that you don't have to give up burgers when you give up bread. These protein-style burgers replace the bread with large pieces of lettuce used as a wrap. Alternatively, you can eat the turkey patty like a steak, with the condiments piled on top or parked beside for dipping.

1 pound ground turkey

½ teaspoon fish sauce

2 garlic cloves, minced

3 drops liquid stevia, or to taste

1 teaspoon sea salt

¼ teaspoon freshly ground black pepper

8 large butter, iceberg, or romaine lettuce leaves

4 tablespoons Pub-Style Burger Sauce (page 227)

1 recipe Caramelized Onions (page 237)

1. Preheat the oven to 375ºF.

2. In a large bowl, combine the ground turkey, fish sauce, garlic, stevia, salt, and pepper. Form into four patties.

3. Place the patties on a rack set over a baking pan. Bake in the preheated oven for 30 minutes, or until the internal temperature of the turkey reaches 170ºF.

4. Put each turkey burger on a piece of lettuce and top with the burger sauce and caramelized onions. Top with a second piece of lettuce.

Variation Tip *If you don't have fish sauce, use Worcestershire or gluten-free soy sauce, both of which add a similar savory flavor to the turkey.*

PER SERVING Calories: 354; Total Fat: 24g; Saturated Fat: 4g; Cholesterol: 119mg; Carbohydrates: 7g; Fiber: <1g; Protein: 32g

TURKEY AND
SPINACH ROULADE

···································

SERVES 4 · PREP TIME: 10 MINUTES · COOK TIME: 30 MINUTES

The title may sound fancy, but this is just turkey breast wrapped around flavorful spinach and baked. Tying the roulade with butcher's twine helps it hold its shape as it bakes, although you can use toothpicks or wooden skewers as well. Just be sure to soak anything wooden in water before you use them with food that's going in the oven.

2 tablespoons extra-virgin olive oil

4 cups baby spinach

¾ teaspoon sea salt, divided

¼ teaspoon freshly ground
  black pepper

3 garlic cloves, minced

1 teaspoon freshly grated lemon zest

1 (1-pound) boneless turkey breast

1. Preheat the oven to 350°F.

2. In a large, nonstick sauté pan over medium-high heat, heat the olive oil until it shimmers.

3. Add the spinach, ½ teaspoon of salt, and the pepper and cook, stirring constantly, for 2 minutes, or until the spinach wilts.

4. Add the garlic and lemon zest and cook, stirring constantly, for 30 seconds. Let cool slightly.

5. Meanwhile, cut the turkey breast into four flat pieces. Put the pieces between two pieces of parchment and pound them with a mallet until they are ¼ inch thick.

6. Season the turkey with the remaining ¼ teaspoon of salt.

7. Spoon equal portions of the spinach onto the turkey pieces. Roll the turkey around the spinach filling and secure with butcher's twine or a toothpick.

8. Put the roulades in a rimmed baking pan. Bake in the preheated oven for 30 minutes or until the internal temperature of the turkey reaches 170ºF and the juices run clear.

Variation Tip *This works with any type of greens you enjoy, such as collard greens or kale. You can also substitute chicken breast for the turkey, or use dark meat cuts rather than breast meat, if you prefer.*

PER SERVING Calories: 189; Total Fat: 9g; Saturated Fat: 1g; Cholesterol: 49mg; Carbohydrates: 7g; Fiber: 1g; Protein: 20g

TURKEY MEATBALLS

SERVES 4 · PREP TIME: 15 MINUTES · COOK TIME: 20 MINUTES

These savory meatballs are equally delicious when made with either turkey or chicken, and they bake quickly. You can save even more time by using a stand mixer to combine the ingredients.

1 pound ground turkey

4 ounces mushrooms, very finely chopped

2 teaspoons chopped fresh dill

3 garlic cloves, minced

1 shallot, minced

1 egg, lightly beaten

1 teaspoon sea salt

⅛ teaspoon freshly ground black pepper

1. Preheat the oven to 350ºF.
2. Line a baking sheet with parchment paper.
3. In a large bowl, mix the turkey, mushrooms, dill, garlic, shallot, egg, salt, and pepper. Roll into golf ball–sized portions and place on the prepared baking sheet.
4. Bake in the preheated oven for about 20 minutes, or until the meatballs are cooked through. Serve.

Cooking Tip *If you have a food processor, finely chopping the mushrooms is very easy. Pulse the mushrooms for 10 one-second pulses.*

PER SERVING Calories: 248; Total Fat: 14g; Saturated fat: 2g; Cholesterol: 157mg; Carbohydrates: 2g; Fiber: 0g; Protein: 34g

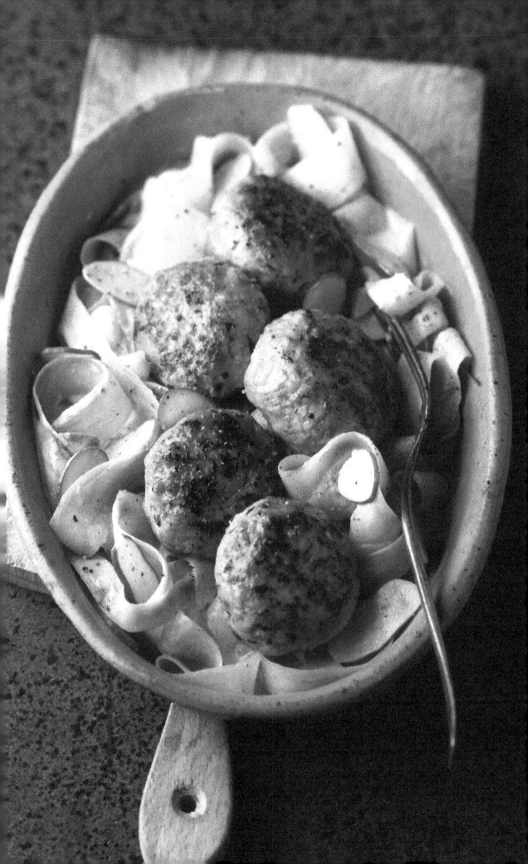

BACON-WRAPPED DRUMSTICKS
WITH ASPARAGUS

....

SERVES 4 · PREP TIME: 10 MINUTES · COOK TIME: 65 MINUTES

I am a huge fan of one-pan meals, because it means less dish-washing and more time to spend with my family. I'm also a huge fan of bacon. As you can probably imagine, that combo makes this one of my favorite quick weeknight recipes—and it's delicious.

2 bunches asparagus, trimmed

12 chicken drumsticks

12 slices thin-cut bacon

1. Preheat the oven to 375°F.
2. Arrange the asparagus in a single layer in the bottom of a 9-by-13-inch baking pan.
3. Wrap each chicken leg in bacon and place on top of the asparagus.
4. Bake in the preheated oven for 65 minutes, or until the chicken juices run clear.

Ingredient Tip Try to find a nitrate-free bacon from pastured pork. I really like the bacon they have at US Wellness Meats online, but many grocery stores, including Trader Joe's, offer other viable options.

PER SERVING Calories: 330; Total Fat: 12g; Saturated Fat: 4g; Cholesterol: 136mg; Carbohydrates: 5g; Fiber: 3g; Protein: 48g

APPLE AND CRANBERRY PORK LOIN

SERVES 6 · PREP TIME: 15 MINUTES
COOK TIME: 65 MINUTES, PLUS 20 MINUTES TO REST

Pork loin is a tasty, lean meat. The earthy flavor of the pork marries beautifully with the pungent herbs, tart cranberries, and sweet apples in this dish.

2 tablespoons coconut oil

3 apples, peeled, cored, and chopped

½ cup dried unsweetened cranberries

1 teaspoon dried sage

1 teaspoon dried rosemary

1½ teaspoons sea salt, divided

¼ teaspoon freshly ground black pepper, divided

1 (3-pound) boneless pork loin, butterflied

1. Preheat the oven to 325ºF.

2. In a large sauté pan over medium-high heat, heat the coconut oil until it shimmers.

3. Add the apples, cranberries, sage, rosemary, 1 teaspoon of salt, and ⅛ teaspoon of pepper. Cook, stirring occasionally, until the apples soften, about 5 minutes.

4. Meanwhile, using a meat mallet, pound the pork to a thickness of ½ inch.Season the pork all over with the remaining ½ teaspoon of salt and ⅛ teaspoon of pepper.

5. Spread the apple mixture evenly onto the cut side of the pork. Roll the pork into a cylinder around the filling and secure it with kitchen twine.

6. Transfer the tenderloin to a roasting pan. Roast in the preheated oven for 1 hour, or until the pork reaches an internal temperature of 145ºF. Let the pork rest for 20 minutes before slicing and serving.

PER SERVING Calories: 641; Total Fat: 36g; Saturated Fat: 16g; Cholesterol: 181mg; Carbohydrates: 14g; Fiber: 3g; Protein: 62g

PORK TENDERLOIN WITH ONIONS, FIGS, AND ROSEMARY

SERVES 6 · PREP TIME: 15 MINUTES
COOK TIME: 40 MINUTES, PLUS 10 MINUTES TO REST

If you find fresh figs in the grocery store, buy them! Most fig trees produce two crops annually, and the fruit is typically available in late spring/early summer and in late summer/early fall. They add a sweetness to the earthy pork in this recipe that is really tasty.

2 (1-pound) pork tenderloins

½ teaspoon sea salt, plus more for seasoning

¼ teaspoon freshly ground black pepper, plus more for seasoning

2 tablespoons extra-virgin olive oil

1 onion, sliced

1 teaspoon dried rosemary

10 fresh figs, quartered

2 tablespoons balsamic vinegar

1. Preheat the oven to 300°F.

2. Season the pork tenderloin with salt and pepper.

3. In a large sauté pan over medium-high heat, heat the olive oil until it shimmers. Add the tenderloins and cook for 3 minutes per side, or until browned all over. Put the tenderloins on a baking sheet.

4. Roast the tenderloins in the preheated oven for 15 minutes, or until the internal temperature reaches 140°F.

5. In the meantime, return the sauté pan to medium-high heat. Add the onions and rosemary and cook, stirring occasionally, for 5 minutes, or until soft. Reduce the heat to low and cook, stirring occasionally, for a further 15 minutes, or until the onions are very browned and starting to caramelize.

6. Add the figs, ½ teaspoon of salt, and ¼ teaspoon of pepper. Cook, stirring frequently, for 5 minutes, or until the figs are soft.

7. Add the balsamic vinegar and use the edge of the spoon to scrape any browned bits from the bottom of the pan. Remove from the heat.

8. Let the tenderloins rest for 10 minutes before slicing. Slice the tenderloins and serve with the onion and fig mixture.

Cooking Tip *The balsamic vinegar is used to deglaze the pan, picking up the bits of flavor stuck to the bottom of the pan. If you don't have balsamic, you can use a little bit of chicken broth or even water instead.*

PER SERVING Calories: 344; Total Fat: 10g; Saturated Fat: 3g; Cholesterol: 110mg; Carbohydrates: 22g; Fiber: 4g; Protein: 41g

PAN-SEARED PORK CHOPS WITH APPLE BUTTER

SERVES 4 · PREP TIME: 5 MINUTES · COOK TIME: 10 MINUTES

Pork chops can be tricky to cook. If you use the wrong method, they can wind up dry. That's because pork chops, although they have fat around the edge, have very little intramuscular fat to keep them moist. For that reason, pan searing is a great choice for pork chops. It seals in the moisture quickly without long exposure to dry heat, which can dry out the chops.

4 boneless, thick-cut pork chops

Sea salt

Freshly ground black pepper

2 tablespoons extra-virgin olive oil

2 tablespoons minced shallots

2 garlic cloves, minced

1 cup Chicken Broth (page 228)

2 cups Apple Butter (page 225)

1. Season the pork chops liberally with salt and pepper.

2. In a large sauté pan over medium-high heat, heat the olive oil until it shimmers. Add the pork chops. Cook without moving for 3 minutes, or until browned on one side. Flip the pork chops and cook for 3 minutes on the other side, or until browned. Set the pork chops aside, tented with foil.

3. To the fat in the pan, add the shallots and cook, stirring occasionally, for 4 minutes, or until soft.

4. Add the garlic and cook, stirring constantly, for 30 seconds, or until fragrant.

5. Add the chicken broth, using the edge of a spoon to scrape any browned bits from the bottom of the pan. Bring to a simmer.

6. Whisk in the apple butter. Bring to a simmer.

7. Return the pork chops to the pan. Turn the chops to coat them with sauce. Serve with the sauce spooned over the pork chops.

Cooking Tip Pan sauces, like the one in this recipe, are really easy to make and add a lot of flavor to quick-seared meats. It's essential that you make the sauce in the same pan that you cooked the meat, and that you deglaze the pan with liquid to get any flavorful browned bits from the bottom of the pan. You can use any liquid to deglaze, and feel free to experiment with herbs and spices to make a tasty sauce.

PER SERVING Calories: 442; Total Fat: 11g; Saturated Fat: 2g; Cholesterol: 60mg; Carbohydrates: 62g; Fiber: 2g; Protein: 23g

ASIAN PORK MEATBALLS WITH GINGERED BOK CHOY

....

SERVES 4 · PREP TIME: 15 MINUTES · COOK TIME: 40 MINUTES

I love meatballs because they are so easy to make, and they're really versatile as far as the flavors you can add. Sometimes I make these alone and serve them with the bok choy, and sometimes I toss them in chicken broth with veggies to make a soup. Feel free to play with the ingredients to give the meatballs your own unique flair.

1½ pounds ground pork

3 teaspoons grated peeled ginger, divided

4 garlic cloves, minced, divided

2 scallions, minced

2 tablespoons chopped fresh cilantro leaves

1½ teaspoons sea salt, divided

2 tablespoons coconut oil

1 head bok choy, chopped

1. Preheat the oven to 400°F. Line a baking sheet with parchment paper.

2. In a large bowl, mix the pork, 2 teaspoons of ginger, 3 garlic cloves, the scallions, cilantro, and 1 teaspoon of salt. Roll into 1-inch balls and put the meatballs on the prepared baking sheet.

3. Bake in the preheated oven for 30 minutes, or until the meatballs are cooked through.

4. Meanwhile, in a large sauté pan over medium-high heat, heat the coconut oil until it shimmers.

5. Add the bok choy and the remaining 1 teaspoon of ginger. Cook, stirring occasionally, for 5 minutes, or until the bok choy is soft and wilted.

6. Add the remaining garlic clove and the remaining ½ teaspoon of salt. Cook, stirring constantly, for 30 seconds, or until fragrant.

7. Serve the meatballs with the bok choy.

Variation Tip *To make meatball soup, bring your favorite broth to a boil. Add vegetables such as shiitake mushrooms and carrots, and then add the formed meatballs. Boil the soup for 30 minutes to cook the meatballs. You can stir in some bok choy in the last 5 minutes.*

PER SERVING Calories: 341; Total Fat: 13g; Saturated Fat: 8g; Cholesterol: 124mg; Carbohydrates: 7g; Fiber: 3g; Protein: 48g

TRI-TIP TACOS

SERVES 4 · PREP TIME: 10 MINUTES, PLUS 2 HOURS TO MARINATE
COOK TIME: 10 MINUTES, PLUS 10 MINUTES TO REST

Tri-tip roast has a really strong beef flavor, so it's especially tasty. It also sears very quickly in a hot sauté pan, so cooking takes no time at all. To speed things up even more, you can marinate the steaks in the morning so they're ready for the pan as soon as you get home. You'll have dinner on the table in about 20 minutes.

6 scallions, chopped

¼ cup chopped fresh cilantro leaves

6 garlic cloves, minced

Zest of 1 lime

¼ cup plus 2 tablespoons extra-virgin olive oil, divided

½ cup apple cider vinegar

1 teaspoon sea salt

1 (1½-pound) tri-tip roast

8 large romaine lettuce leaves

1 recipe Guacamole (page 234)

1. In a blender or food processor, combine the scallions, cilantro, garlic, lime zest, ¼ cup of olive oil, apple cider vinegar, and sea salt. Blend on high speed until smooth.

2. Set aside 2 tablespoons of the mixture. Pour the remaining marinade into a large zipper-close bag and add the tri-tip roast. Squish the roast around in the sealed bag to distribute the marinade. Refrigerate for at least 2 hours and as many as 12 hours.

3. In a large sauté pan over medium-high heat, heat the remaining 2 tablespoons of olive oil until it shimmers.

4. Wipe the excess marinade off the roast and sear it in the pan for 4 minutes per side.

5. Let the meat rest for 10 minutes.

6. Cut the steak on the bias into strips. Toss the strips with the reserved 2 tablespoons of marinade mixture.

7. Spoon onto the lettuce leaves and top with the guacamole.

PER SERVING Calories: 585; Total Fat: 42g; Saturated Fat: 9g; Cholesterol: 121mg; Carbohydrates: 8g; Fiber: 3g; Protein: 48g

SLOW COOKER BEEF STEW WITH FENNEL AND MUSHROOMS

SERVES 4 · PREP TIME: 10 MINUTES · COOK TIME: 8 HOURS, 30 MINUTES

Fennel and mushrooms are one of my favorite flavor combos. Beef stew meat is flavorful, but it tends to be really tough unless you cook it low and slow with moist heat, which is why it is ideal for your slow cooker. Cooking it under these conditions keeps the meat moist, and the long, slow cooking temperature allows the collagen in the meat to break down and soften. Serve with mashed sweet potatoes or cooked brown rice.

1½ pounds beef stew meat

1 red onion, chopped

1 fennel bulb, chopped

1 pound cremini mushrooms, quartered

1 teaspoon mustard powder

1 teaspoon garlic powder

1 teaspoon dried thyme

1 teaspoon sea salt

½ teaspoon freshly ground black pepper

4 cups Chicken or Beef Broth (page 228), divided

2 tablespoons arrowroot powder

1. In a large slow cooker, combine the stew meat, red onion, fennel, mushrooms, mustard powder, garlic powder, thyme, salt, pepper, and 3 cups of chicken or beef broth.

2. Cover the slow cooker and set it on low. Cook for 8 hours.

3. About 30 minutes before dinner, turn the slow cooker up to high, and remove the lid. In a small bowl, whisk together the arrowroot powder and the remaining 1 cup broth. Stir it into the stew. Simmer for another 30 minutes.

Variation Tip You don't have to limit yourself to beef for this stew. Try other cuts of meat, such as pork shoulder (cut into cubes), game meats, or even chicken thighs. If you have a tough but fatty cut of meat on your hands, this stew is just the ticket for a delicious meal.

PER SERVING Calories: 723; Total Fat: 27g; Saturated Fat: 10g; Cholesterol: 288mg; Carbohydrates: 17g; Fiber: 3g; Protein: 98g

POT ROAST WITH
SWEET POTATOES AND SHALLOTS

SERVES 8 · PREP TIME: 15 MINUTES · COOK TIME: 3 HOURS

Chuck roast is an affordable cut of meat, but you have to cook it under the right conditions so it's nice and tender. Pot roast is essentially a braise that is cooked low and slow with plenty of liquid—the perfect conditions for softening up tough chuck roast. All you have to do while the roast cooks is sit back and relax.

2 tablespoons extra-virgin olive oil

1 (3-pound) chuck roast

Sea salt

Freshly ground black pepper

6 shallots, peeled and quartered

2 sweet potatoes, peeled and cubed

½ cup red wine vinegar

3½ cups Beef Broth (page 228)

1 teaspoon garlic powder

1 teaspoon dried thyme

1. Preheat the oven to 275°F.

2. In a Dutch oven over medium-high heat, heat the olive oil until it shimmers.

3. Season the roast liberally with salt and pepper. Sear the pot roast on all sides by cooking for 3 minutes per side, or until browned.

4. Remove the roast and set aside. Add the shallots and sweet potatoes to the pan and cook, stirring occasionally, for 5 minutes, or until they start to brown.

5. Add the red wine vinegar and use a wooden spoon to scrape any browned bits from the bottom of the pan.

6. Add the beef broth, garlic powder, and dried thyme. Return the roast to the pan, arranging the vegetables around it. Bring to a simmer.

7. Cover the Dutch oven and transfer it to the preheated oven. Cook for 3 hours, or until the meat is very tender.

PER SERVING Calories: 502; Total Fat: 18g; Saturated Fat: 6g; Cholesterol: 172mg; Carbohydrates: 20g; Fiber: 2g; Protein: 60g

GROUND BEEF AND
ASPARAGUS STIR-FRY

SERVES 4 · PREP TIME: 10 MINUTES · COOK TIME: 10 MINUTES

This is a super easy stir-fry that's high in iron, protein, copper, and selenium. It's also pretty tasty and freezes well for meals on the go. Experiment by adding any veggies or seasonings you wish to really make this stir-fry shine.

1 pound ground beef

1 red onion, chopped

12 asparagus spears, trimmed and chopped

8 ounces cremini mushrooms, sliced

2 garlic cloves, minced

2 tablespoons Worcestershire sauce

1 tablespoon Dijon mustard

½ cup Chicken Broth (page 228)

1 tablespoon arrowroot powder

2 cups cooked brown rice

1. In a large sauté pan over medium-high heat, cook the ground beef, crumbling with a spoon, for 5 minutes, or until browned.

2. Add the onion, asparagus, and mushrooms and cook, stirring frequently, for 5 minutes, or until the vegetables are tender.

3. Add the garlic and cook, stirring constantly, for 30 seconds, or until fragrant.

4. Meanwhile, in a small bowl, whisk together the Worcestershire sauce, Dijon mustard, chicken broth, and arrowroot powder until smooth.

5. Add the sauce to the pan. Cook, stirring constantly, until the meat and vegetables are coated with the sauce.

6. Serve spooned over brown rice.

Ingredient Tip Arrowroot is a tuber that is processed into a powder to thicken soups and sauces. It works in a manner similar to cornstarch. When working with arrowroot, you always want to make a slurry by whisking it into a liquid before adding it to the pan; otherwise, you'll wind up with a lumpy sauce.

PER SERVING Calories: 618; Total Fat: 10g; Saturated Fat: 3g; Cholesterol: 101mg; Carbohydrates: 84g; Fiber: 6g; Protein: 45g

GYRO SALAD

SERVES 8 · PREP TIME: 15 MINUTES · COOK TIME: 1 HOUR, PLUS 10 MINUTES TO REST

Most commercial gyros contain breadcrumbs. Since I love gyros, I knew I had to come up with my own gluten-free version. This one is gluten-free, Paleo, and low in carbohydrates, but it remains true to the original flavor of gyros as well.

1 onion, grated	2 pounds ground lamb
8 garlic cloves, minced	12 cups arugula
2 teaspoons dried rosemary	1 recipe Pickled Red Onions (page 236)
1 teaspoon sea salt	¼ cup Basil Vinaigrette (page 230)
½ teaspoon freshly ground black pepper	¼ cup Easy Mayonnaise (page 235)

1. Preheat the oven to 325°F.
2. Wrap the grated onion in a tea towel and twist it over the sink to wring the water out of the onions. Put the onions, garlic, rosemary, salt, pepper, and lamb in a blender, food processor, or stand mixer. Blend on high speed for 3 minutes, or until the ingredients almost resemble a paste.
3. Press the mixture into a loaf pan.
4. Pour enough boiling water into a 9-by-13-inch baking pan to come halfway up the sides. Put the filled loaf pan in the water bath, and carefully transfer the pans to the oven.
5. Bake for 1 hour, or until the internal temperature is 165°F.
6. Let the meat rest for 10 minutes. Slice thinly.
7. Arrange the meat on a bed of arugula and top with the pickled red onions.
8. In a small bowl, whisk together the basil vinaigrette and the mayonnaise. Toss with the salad.

PER SERVING Calories: 299; Total Fat: 15g; Saturated Fat: 4g; Cholesterol: 104mg; Carbohydrates: 7g; Fiber: 1g; Protein: 33g

HERB-RUBBED LEG OF LAMB

SERVES 10 · PREP TIME: 15 MINUTES
COOK TIME: 1 HOUR, 15 MINUTES, PLUS 10 MINUTES TO REST

This makes a lot, because there's not really any such thing as a small leg of lamb. However, it works really well for a crowd, and you can freeze the cooked meat in single-serving portions to use for meals on the go, or to top a tasty salad. Serve with Cucumber Salad with Ginger-Cilantro Vinaigrette (page 157) or Apple-Ginger Slaw (page 162).

¼ cup fresh rosemary leaves

1 bunch fresh chives, chopped

½ cup loosely packed fresh basil leaves

6 garlic cloves, minced

2 tablespoons extra-virgin olive oil

1 teaspoon sea salt

½ teaspoon freshly ground black pepper

2 tablespoons Dijon mustard

1 (5-pound) bone-in leg of lamb

1. Preheat the oven to 400°F.

2. In a food processor or blender, combine the rosemary, chives, basil, garlic, olive oil, salt, pepper, and mustard. Process for 1 minute, or until smooth.

3. Put the lamb in a Dutch oven.

4. Rub the herb mixture over the surface of the lamb. Roast, uncovered, in the preheated oven for 20 minutes.

5. Reduce the oven temperature to 300°F and continue to roast for another 55 minutes, or until the internal temperature of the lamb reaches 145°F.

6. Let the lamb rest for 10 minutes before carving.

Cooking Tip If you're using a food processor, you don't need to mince any of the ingredients. However, if you're using a blender, do mince all of the ingredients before combining them.

PER SERVING Calories: 456; Total Fat: 20g; Saturated Fat: 7g; Cholesterol: 204mg; Carbohydrates: 2g; Fiber: <1g; Protein: 64g

12

FISH AND SHELLFISH DINNERS

PAN-SEARED COD WITH ROASTED BUTTERNUT SQUASH

....

SERVES 4 · PREP TIME: 15 MINUTES · COOK TIME: 30 MINUTES

Season the butternut squash with a bit of cumin to enhance its sweet flavors. Nicely caramelized cubes of sweet and earthy squash make the perfect accompaniment to simple pan-seared cod fillets flavored with a hint of coriander and lime zest.

1 butternut squash, peeled, seeded, and cut into 1-inch cubes

4 tablespoons extra-virgin olive oil, divided

1 teaspoon ground cumin, divided

1 teaspoon sea salt, divided

½ teaspoon freshly ground black pepper, divided

1 teaspoon ground coriander

1 teaspoon freshly grated lime zest

4 (4- to 6-ounce) cod fillets

½ cup Guacamole (page 234)

1. Preheat the oven to 425°F.

2. In a large bowl, toss the squash with 2 tablespoons of olive oil, ½ teaspoon of cumin, ½ teaspoon of salt, and ¼ teaspoon of black pepper.

3. Put the squash in a single layer on a large baking sheet and roast in the preheated oven for 30 minutes, or until it begins to brown.

4. Meanwhile, in a large sauté pan over medium-high heat, heat the remaining 2 tablespoons of olive oil until it shimmers.

5. In a small bowl, combine the remaining ½ teaspoon of cumin, remaining ½ teaspoon of salt, remaining ¼ teaspoon of pepper, the coriander, and the lime zest. Sprinkle liberally over the cod fillets.

6. Place the cod flesh-side down in the pan and cook for 5 minutes. Flip the cod and cook for 5 minutes, or until the flesh is flaky and opaque.

7. Serve the cod, topped with guacamole, alongside the butternut squash.

PER SERVING Calories: 305; Total Fat: 21g; Saturated Fat: 3g; Cholesterol: 62mg; Carbohydrates: 4g; Fiber: 2g; Protein: 27g

ROASTED HALIBUT
WITH DILL AND ZUCCHINI

SERVES 4 · PREP TIME: 15 MINUTES · COOK TIME: 12 MINUTES

Halibut has a sweet, delicate flesh that is simply delicious. Adding the classic flavor of dill and combining it with zucchini in a single pan makes preparation and cleanup of this meal a snap. It's a good summertime meal because it is so light and delicate, but you can enjoy it any time of year.

1 teaspoon dried dill

1 teaspoon freshly grated lemon zest

1 teaspoon sea salt

⅛ teaspoon freshly ground black pepper

4 (4- to 6-ounce) halibut fillets

2 zucchini, chopped

2 tablespoons extra-virgin olive oil

1. Preheat the oven to 500°F.
2. In a small bowl, combine the dill, lemon zest, salt, and pepper.
3. Sprinkle half of the mixture on the halibut and place the fillets flesh-side up in a large baking pan.
4. In a large bowl, toss the zucchini with the remaining spice mixture and the olive oil.
5. Arrange the zucchini around the halibut.
6. Roast in the preheated oven for 10 minutes, or until the zucchini is soft and the fish is cooked.

Variation Tip Dill works with most fish. Try this with a fattier fish, such as salmon, for a different flavor and texture. You can also use other varieties of summer squash, such as yellow squash or pattypan squash.

PER SERVING Calories: 196; Total Fat: 8g; Saturated Fat: 1g; Cholesterol: 62mg; Carbohydrates: 4g; Fiber: 1g; Protein: 27g

GINGER-SOY SALMON WITH SAUTÉED SPINACH

....

SERVES 4 · PREP TIME: 15 MINUTES, PLUS 10 MINUTES TO MARINATE
COOK TIME: 15 MINUTES

This dish is as easy as it comes, and it only dirties one pan—another snappy-cleanup dish. I've lived in the Pacific Northwest my entire life, so salmon is always on the menu, which has encouraged me to create dozens of ways to prepare it.

¼ cup gluten-free soy sauce or tamari

¼ cup Chicken Broth (page 228)

1 tablespoon peeled grated ginger

3 garlic cloves, minced, divided

2 teaspoons freshly grated
  lime zest, divided

4 (4- to 6-ounce) salmon fillets

2 tablespoons coconut oil

4 cups baby spinach

¼ teaspoon sea salt

¼ teaspoon freshly ground
  black pepper

1. In a large bowl, whisk together the soy sauce, chicken broth, ginger, 2 minced garlic cloves, and 1 teaspoon of lime zest. Add the salmon and let it marinate for 10 minutes.

2. In a large sauté pan over medium-high heat, heat the coconut oil until it shimmers. Add the salmon, flesh-side down, and cook for 3 minutes. Flip the salmon and cook for 5 minutes, or until the flesh flakes easily with a fork. Remove the salmon from the pan and set aside on a plate.

3. Add the spinach, the remaining 1 teaspoon of lime zest, the salt, and the pepper to the pan and cook, stirring occasionally, for 2 minutes, or until the spinach wilts.

4. Add the remaining 1 minced garlic clove and cook, stirring constantly, for 30 seconds, or until fragrant.

5. Serve the spinach alongside the salmon fillets.

PER SERVING Calories: 206; Total Fat: 9g; Saturated Fat: 1g; Cholesterol: 63mg; Carbohydrates: 3g; Fiber: 1g; Protein: 29g

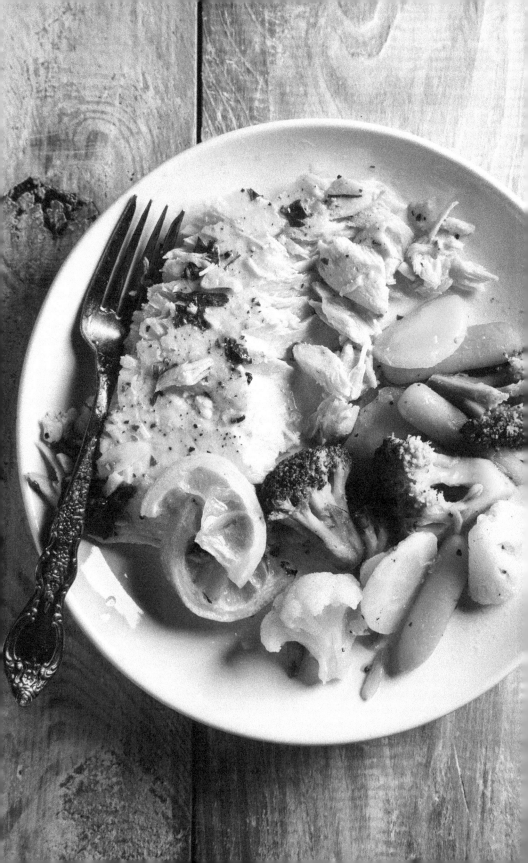

SALMON AND VEGETABLES IN FOIL PACKETS

....

SERVES 4 · PREP TIME: 10 MINUTES · COOK TIME: 40 MINUTES

Cooking salmon wrapped in foil packets makes it super moist. Adding the vegetables to the packets allows them to steam as the salmon cooks, giving you bright, tender-crisp vegetables.

4 (6-ounce) salmon fillets

2 golden beets, peeled and chopped

2 cups broccoli florets

2 cups cauliflower florets

16 baby carrots

¼ cup extra-virgin olive oil

1 teaspoon dried tarragon

1 teaspoon sea salt

¼ teaspoon freshly ground black pepper

1 cup Chicken Broth (page 228)

1. Preheat the oven to 400°F.

2. Cut four sheets of foil into 17-inch lengths. Fold the edges of each length of foil upward to make a bowl that you can seal on top. Place the foil bowls on a rimmed baking sheet.

3. Place a salmon fillet in each foil bowl and arrange the beets, broccoli, cauliflower, and baby carrots around the salmon.

4. Drizzle the salmon and vegetables with the olive oil. Sprinkle with the tarragon, salt, and pepper.

5. Divide the chicken broth evenly among the packets, pouring it in along the edges of the fish and veggies.

6. Carefully wrap the sides of the foil inward and tightly seal the packets around the salmon and vegetables. Bake in the pre-heated oven for about 40 minutes, or until the salmon flakes easily with a fork.

Variation Tip If you like lemon, squeeze a wedge of lemon over each packet and then add the squeezed lemon wedges to the packet before sealing.

PER SERVING Calories: 397; Total Fat: 25g; Saturated Fat: 4g; Cholesterol: 75mg; Carbohydrates: 9g; Fiber: 4g; Protein: 37g

GARLIC SHRIMP WITH SPAGHETTI SQUASH

·····························

SERVES 4 · PREP TIME: 15 MINUTES · COOK TIME: 40 MINUTES

Spaghetti squash is an excellent stand-in for pasta—in this, and many other pasta dishes. It's easy to prepare in the oven. This recipe walks you through the steps. We've topped our version with sautéed shrimp, but you can also enjoy spaghetti squash with your favorite pasta sauce.

1 spaghetti squash, halved pole-to-pole and seeded

3 tablespoons extra-virgin olive oil

1½ pounds medium shrimp, peeled, deveined, and tails removed

6 garlic cloves, minced

1 teaspoon freshly grated lemon zest

1 teaspoon sea salt

¼ teaspoon freshly ground black pepper

¼ cup chopped fresh parsley leaves

1. Preheat the oven to 375°F.

2. Put the squash halves on a baking sheet, cut-side down. Bake for 40 minutes, or until soft.

3. Meanwhile, in a large sauté pan over medium-high heat, heat the olive oil until it shimmers.

4. Add the shrimp and cook, stirring occasionally, for 4 minutes, or until the shrimp turns pink.

5. Add the garlic, lemon zest, salt, and pepper. Cook, stirring constantly, for 30 seconds, or until the garlic is fragrant. Remove from the heat and stir in the parsley.

6. Using a fork, scrape the flesh of the roasted spaghetti squash to create strands. Serve the squash topped with the shrimp.

Ingredient Tip While you can take the time to peel and devein the shrimp, it's pretty easy to find it already done for you. Look in the frozen seafood section of your favorite grocery store.

PER SERVING Calories: 284; Total Fat: 13g; Saturated Fat: 2g; Cholesterol: 334mg; Carbohydrates: 7g; Fiber: 0g; Protein: 37g

TURMERIC SHRIMP-STUFFED SWEET POTATOES

SERVES 4 · PREP TIME: 10 MINUTES · COOK TIME: 45 MINUTES

Turmeric is anti-inflammatory and an excellent source of antioxidants. Its golden color makes the shrimp visually interesting, and the turmeric adds a delicious sharp, spicy flavor to the dish. Stuffing the potatoes with the shrimp moistens the flesh of the potatoes for a delicious dinner.

4 tablespoons coconut oil, divided

4 small sweet potatoes, washed and pierced several times with a fork

1 onion, chopped

1 teaspoon ground turmeric

1 pound shrimp, peeled, deveined, and tails removed

1 teaspoon sea salt

¼ teaspoon freshly ground black pepper

1. Preheat the oven to 400°F.

2. Using a paper towel, rub 2 tablespoons of coconut oil on the outside of the sweet potatoes.

3. Put the potatoes on a baking sheet and bake in the preheated oven for 45 minutes, or until soft.

4. Meanwhile, in a large sauté pan over medium-high heat, heat the remaining 2 tablespoons of coconut oil until the oil shimmers.

5. Add the onion and turmeric and cook, stirring occasionally, for 4 minutes, or until the onion is soft and the turmeric is fragrant.

6. Add the shrimp, salt, and pepper. Cook, stirring occasionally, for 4 minutes, or until the shrimp is cooked through.

7. To serve, split open the cooked sweet potatoes and spoon on the shrimp.

Variation Tip *Replace the turmeric with ground cinnamon, another healthy spice that works really well with shrimp and sweet potatoes.*

PER SERVING Calories: 442; Total Fat: 16g; Saturated Fat: 12g; Cholesterol: 239mg; Carbohydrates: 47g; Fiber: 7g; Protein: 29g

PAN-SEARED SCALLOPS WITH ROASTED GREEN BEANS AND GARLIC AIOLI

SERVES 4 · PREP TIME: 15 MINUTES · COOK TIME: 25 MINUTES

Roasting green beans is a great way to add extra flavor because high-heat roasting caramelizes the outside of the vegetables. Likewise, pan-seared scallops develop a flavorful dark crust. Drizzling both with garlic aïoli brings the flavors together beautifully.

1 pound green beans, trimmed

4 tablespoons extra-virgin olive oil, divided

1 teaspoon sea salt, divided

½ teaspoon freshly ground black pepper, divided

1½ pounds sea scallops

½ cup Easy Mayonnaise (page 235)

2 tablespoons red wine vinegar

2 garlic cloves, minced

1. Preheat the oven to 400°F.

2. In a large bowl, toss the green beans with 2 tablespoons of olive oil, ½ teaspoon of salt, and ¼ teaspoon of black pepper. Put the beans in a 9-by-13-inch baking pan in a single layer.

3. Roast the green beans in the preheated oven for 25 minutes, or until caramelized and cooked through.

4. Meanwhile, pat the scallops dry with paper towels. Season them on both sides with the remaining ½ teaspoon of salt and ¼ teaspoon of pepper.

5. In a large sauté pan over medium-high heat, heat the remaining 2 tablespoons of olive oil until it shimmers.

6. Add the scallops, searing them on one side for 2 minutes, or until browned, then turning and doing the same on the other side.

7. In a small bowl, whisk together the mayonnaise, red wine vinegar, and garlic.

8. To serve, drizzle the garlic aïoli over the scallops and green beans.

Ingredient Tip *Scallops have a muscle attached to the side that becomes tough when cooked. Use a sharp paring knife to carefully cut it away before cooking.*

PER SERVING Calories: 424; Total Fat: 25g; Saturated Fat: 4g; Cholesterol: 64mg; Carbohydrates: 20g; Fiber: 4g; Protein: 31g

SEA SCALLOP GREMOLATA WITH ROASTED BABY CARROTS

································

SERVES 4 · PREP TIME: 15 MINUTES · COOK TIME: 25 MINUTES

Gremolata is really easy to make and adds a depth of freshness and flavor to the scallops in this dish. Searing the scallops takes only minutes, while using baby carrots eliminates peeling and chopping time. Using your blender or food processor to make the gremolata also speeds up prep time.

1 pound baby carrots

4 tablespoons extra-virgin olive oil, divided

1½ teaspoons sea salt, divided

½ teaspoon freshly ground black pepper, divided

1½ pounds sea scallops

¼ cup chopped fresh parsley leaves

4 garlic cloves, minced

Zest of 1 orange

1. Preheat the oven to 425°F.
2. In a large bowl, toss the baby carrots with 2 tablespoons of olive oil, ½ teaspoon of salt, and ¼ teaspoon of black pepper. Put the carrots in a 9-by-13-inch baking pan in a single layer.
3. Roast the carrots in the preheated oven for 25 minutes, or until caramelized and cooked through.
4. Meanwhile, pat the scallops dry with paper towels. Season them on both sides with ½ teaspoon of salt and the remaining ¼ teaspoon of pepper.
5. In a large sauté pan over medium-high heat, heat the remaining 2 tablespoons of olive oil until it shimmers.

6. Add the scallops, searing them on one side for 2 minutes, or until browned, then turning and doing the same on the other side.

7. In a blender or food processor, combine the parsley, garlic, orange zest, and remaining ½ teaspoon of salt.

8. Using 1-second pulses, pulse five to ten times to finely chop the mixture.

9. Serve the scallops and carrots with the gremolata sprinkled over the top.

Variation Tip *You can substitute any type of citrus zest in place of the orange zest. Gremolata is also delicious stirred into stews and soups after they are done cooking.*

PER SERVING Calories: 316; Total Fat: 16g; Saturated Fat: 2g; Cholesterol: 56mg; Carbohydrates: 15g; Fiber: 4g; Protein: 30g

CRAB AND FENNEL SALAD WITH AVOCADO

....

SERVES 4 · PREP TIME: 10 MINUTES · COOK TIME: NONE

This simple salad combines sweet, briny crab with creamy avocado and the crisp bite of fennel. The flavors marry together beautifully, making this a simple yet delicious light summer supper. You can also make it ahead of time and take it for lunch on the go, or even try it as a tasty, yet different breakfast.

12 ounces lump crabmeat, rinsed and picked over for shells

1 fennel bulb, finely chopped

½ red onion, finely chopped

1 avocado, peeled, pitted, and cubed

1 teaspoon freshly grated lemon zest

2 tablespoons finely chopped fennel fronds

½ teaspoon sea salt

¼ teaspoon freshly ground black pepper

½ cup Easy Mayonnaise (page 235)

1. In a large bowl, toss together the crabmeat, fennel, onion, avocado, lemon zest, fennel fronds, salt, and pepper.

2. Gently fold in the mayonnaise. Serve immediately.

Variation Tip *If you can't find crab, or if it's too expensive, you can substitute baby bay shrimp.*

PER SERVING Calories: 303; Total Fat: 27g; Saturated Fat: 4g; Cholesterol: 56mg; Carbohydrates: 18g; Fiber: 6g; Protein: 15g

CRAB CAKES WITH
APPLE-GINGER SLAW
....

SERVES 4 · PREP TIME: 10 MINUTES · COOK TIME: 12 MINUTES

Living in the Pacific Northwest, I'm a huge fan of crab, but traditional crab cakes use breadcrumbs as a binder. I found a way around that, leaving the breadcrumbs out altogether and flavoring the cakes with tasty chopped scallions and grated ginger.

1 pound lump crabmeat, rinsed and picked over for shells

2 teaspoons grated peeled ginger

2 garlic cloves, minced

4 scallions, minced

¾ teaspoon sea salt

¼ teaspoon freshly ground black pepper

1 egg, beaten

¼ cup Easy Mayonnaise (page 235)

1 teaspoon mustard powder

1 recipe Apple-Ginger Slaw (page 162)

1. Preheat the oven to 350°F. Line a baking sheet with parchment paper.

2. In a large bowl, combine the crabmeat, ginger, garlic, scallions, salt, and pepper, mixing well.

3. In a small bowl, whisk together the egg, mayonnaise, and mustard powder. Carefully fold the mixture into the crab mixture.

4. Scoop the mixture into golf ball–sized mounds, squeeze out any excess water, and place the balls 1 inch apart on the prepared baking sheet. Lightly flatten the mounds.

5. Bake in the preheated oven for 12 minutes. Remove from the oven and leave on the baking sheet for 5 minutes before moving the crab cakes to plates.

6. Serve with the apple-ginger slaw.

Ingredient Tip *Lump crabmeat often winds up with little bits of shell in it. To find and remove any shells, put the crabmeat in a colander in the sink and gently and thoroughly pick through it with your fingers.*

PER SERVING Calories: 374; Total Fat: 26g; Saturated Fat: 3g; Cholesterol: 109mg; Carbohydrates: 36g; Fiber: 11g; Protein: 20g

13

SAUCES, DRESSINGS, AND CONDIMENTS

APPLE BUTTER

....

Apple butter is just super-reduced, super-smooth applesauce. I like to use a combination of Granny Smith apples (or another tart green apple) and Honeycrisp apples (or another sweet-tart apple such as Pink Lady) to give the flavor a bit of complexity. Apple butter is wonderful stirred into oats, spread on pancakes or waffles, or even served with pork.

3 Granny Smith apples, peeled, cored, and sliced

3 Honeycrisp apples, peeled, cored, and sliced

3 teaspoons ground cinnamon

⅓ cup apple cider vinegar

1 teaspoon grated peeled ginger

1. In a slow cooker, combine all of the ingredients. Cover and cook on low for 8 hours or high for 4 hours, stirring occasionally.

2. Mash the apples with a potato masher, and then put them in a blender. Blend on high speed for 2 minutes, or until very smooth.

3. Return the apples to the slow cooker. Cook on high, uncovered, stirring occasionally, for 1 to 2 hours more to evaporate the liquid.

4. Store in a covered container in the refrigerator for up to 1 week or in the freezer for up to 1 year.

Variation Tip Feel free to play around with spices that you like. Spices that go well with apples include fennel, nutmeg, and cloves.

PER ½ CUP Calories: 101; Total Fat: <1g; Saturated Fat: 0g; Cholesterol: 0mg; Carbohydrates: 26g; Fiber: 5g; Protein: <1g

BERRY SAUCE

....

YIELD: ½ CUP · PREP TIME: 5 MINUTES · COOK TIME: 10 MINUTES

You can use berry sauce for a number of applications, from adding it to dairy-free yogurt or ice cream to topping fish or poultry. Make this ahead of time and keep it frozen in ice cube trays so you have single servings readily available to thaw.

2 cups mixed berries (fresh or frozen) ½ teaspoon ground cinnamon

¼ cup of water   3 drops liquid stevia

1. Combine all of the ingredients in a large pot and bring to a simmer over medium-high heat.
2. Cook, stirring occasionally, until the berries are soft, about 10 minutes.
3. Transfer the mixture to a blender and blend on high for 30 seconds.
4. Strain the berry sauce through a colander, discarding the seeds and solids.

Ingredient Tip For the most flavorful results, use fresh, seasonal, locally available berries.

PER 2 TABLESPOONS Calories: 31; Total Fat: 0g; Saturated Fat: 0g; Cholesterol: 0mg; Carbohydrates: 8g; Fiber: 2g; Protein: 1g

PUB-STYLE BURGER SAUCE

YIELD: 1 CUP · PREP TIME: 5 MINUTES · COOK TIME: NONE

This is a family favorite at the Frazier house. We love slapping this on turkey and ground beef burgers. The savory flavor takes them to the next level. It's also super easy to make, and the flavor payoff is well worth the five minutes you spend in the kitchen making it.

1 cup Easy Mayonnaise (page 235)

1 tablespoon gluten-free soy sauce or tamari

1 tablespoon Worcestershire sauce

1 garlic clove, minced

2 drops liquid stevia

2 tablespoons chopped fresh chives

1. In a small bowl, combine all of the ingredients.
2. Store, tightly sealed, in the refrigerator for up to 4 days.

Ingredient Tip To make mincing garlic a snap, try a garlic press. I love mine. All I have to do is stick an unpeeled clove of garlic in it, squeeze the handle, and poof: minced garlic! I've tried various presses, but the one that works best for me is the Zyliss model.

PER 2 TABLESPOONS Calories: 138; Total Fat: 15g; Saturated Fat: 2g; Cholesterol: 26mg; Carbohydrates: 2g; Fiber: <1g; Protein: <1g

POULTRY, BEEF, OR VEGETABLE STOCK

....

YIELD: 8 CUPS · PREP TIME: 15 MINUTES · COOK TIME: 3 TO 24 HOURS

One of the best things you can do for the flavor of your foods is to make your own stock. While it may sound time consuming or complicated, it is, in fact, extremely simple. I cook mine in my slow cooker for 24 hours, and there's seldom a time that I don't have stock simmering. You can make it and freeze it for later use in soups, stews, and other recipes. Making stock is a good way to use things you'd normally throw away, like vegetable trimmings and bones from chicken, turkey, or beef that you've cooked.

For Poultry or Beef Stock

Poultry or beef bones such as chicken carcasses, marrow bones, or other bones

1 onion, unpeeled and quartered

2 carrots, unpeeled and cut into three pieces

2 celery stalks, cut into pieces

2 fresh rosemary or thyme sprigs

10 peppercorns

1 teaspoon sea salt

9 cups water

For Vegetable Stock

2 onions, unpeeled and quartered

3 carrots, unpeeled and cut into three pieces

3 celery stalks, cut into pieces

8 ounces fresh mushrooms

2 fresh rosemary or thyme sprigs

10 peppercorns

1 teaspoon sea salt

9 cups water

In a slow cooker

1. In a large slow cooker, combine all of the ingredients.

2. Cover the slow cooker and set it on low. Simmer for 12 to 24 hours.

3. Using a fine-mesh sieve, strain the stock into a bowl. Cover and refrigerate overnight.

4. Skim any fat from the stock and discard it. Store the stock in a covered container in the refrigerator for up to 5 days or in the freezer for up to 12 months.

In a stockpot on the stovetop

1. In a large stockpot, combine all of the ingredients.

2. Bring the liquid to a simmer over medium heat. Reduce the heat to low and simmer for 3 hours.

3. Using a fine-mesh sieve, strain the stock into a bowl. Cover and refrigerate overnight.

4. Skim any fat from the stock and discard it. Store the stock in a covered container in the refrigerator for up to 5 days or in the freezer for up to 12 months.

Cooking Tip   I don't actually add any whole vegetables to my stock. Instead, I keep a large zipper-close bag in my freezer to which I add all my vegetable trimmings as I cook throughout the week. Then, when I'm ready to make stock, I just dump the bag of frozen trimmings into the slow cooker with the herbs, salt, peppercorns, bones (or no bones, for vegetable stock), and water. If you do this, be sure you don't use any strongly flavored vegetables like broccoli or bell peppers, which will impart off-flavors to the stock. I tend to use peels and trimmings from onions, carrots, celery, leeks, fennel, and mushrooms. I also keep a separate large zipper-close bag full of saved bones from meals— chicken, beef, poultry, pork, and any other bones I can get my hands on.

PER 1 CUP Calories: 10; Total Fat: <1g; Saturated Fat: 0g; Cholesterol: 0mg; Carbohydrates: <1g; Fiber: 0g; Protein: <1g

BASIL VINAIGRETTE

YIELD: 1 CUP · PREP TIME: 5 MINUTES · COOK TIME: NONE

Basil adds a fresh, bright flavor to dishes with its minty bite. Be sure to use fresh basil—it loses a lot of its flavor when dried. This dressing is delicious on salads and also makes a great marinade for fish or poultry. Store it in a covered container in the refrigerator for up to 3 weeks. Just give it a whisking before use.

¾ cup extra-virgin olive oil

¼ cup apple cider vinegar

6 garlic cloves, minced

3 tablespoons chopped fresh basil leaves

½ teaspoon Dijon mustard

¼ teaspoon sea salt

⅛ teaspoon freshly ground black pepper

1 drop liquid stevia, or to taste

1. In a small bowl, combine all of the ingredients.
2. Whisk to combine.

Cooking Tip Oil and vinegar don't normally or naturally mix. When making vinaigrettes, mustard acts as an emulsifier to help hold the oil and vinegar together. Even so, you'll still need to whisk or shake your vinaigrette before each use, although it won't separate once tossed with your salad.

PER 2 TABLESPOONS Calories: 167; Total Fat: 19g; Saturated Fat: 3g; Cholesterol: 0mg; Carbohydrates: <1g; Fiber: 0g; Protein: <1g

GINGER-CILANTRO VINAIGRETTE

....

YIELD: 1 CUP · PREP TIME: 5 MINUTES · COOK TIME: NONE

This vinaigrette has an Asian flavor profile, so it works well with chopped salads or as a marinade for fish, beef, pork, or poultry. I really like it combined with cucumbers, because the slight sweetness and refreshing character of the cucumbers contrast beautifully with the bite of the ginger.

¾ cup extra-virgin olive oil

¼ cup apple cider vinegar

3 garlic cloves, minced

3 tablespoons chopped fresh cilantro leaves

1 tablespoon grated peeled ginger

¼ teaspoon freshly grated orange zest

½ teaspoon Dijon mustard

¼ teaspoon sea salt

⅛ teaspoon freshly ground black pepper

1. In a small bowl, combine all of the ingredients.
2. Whisk to combine.

Cooking Tip *The best tool to use for zesting citrus is a rasp-style grater. Run it lightly along the peel, taking only the colored part and leaving the bitter white pith behind.*

PER 2 TABLESPOONS Calories: 167; Total Fat: 19g; Saturated Fat: 3g; Cholesterol: 0mg; Carbohydrates: <1g; Fiber: 0g; Protein: <1g

CHIMICHURRI

YIELD: 1¼ CUPS · PREP TIME: 5 MINUTES · COOK TIME: NONE

This intensely flavored (and colored!) sauce is traditionally served spooned over red meats, such as steak, but it is also delicious on fish or poultry. Chimichurri is a go-to condiment in my kitchen, and I keep discovering new uses.

1 bunch fresh parsley

¼ cup fresh oregano leaves

8 garlic cloves

¾ cup extra-virgin olive oil

¼ cup apple cider vinegar

Zest of 2 lemons

½ teaspoon Dijon mustard

½ teaspoon sea salt

¼ teaspoon freshly ground black pepper

1. In the bowl of a food processor or blender, combine all of the ingredients and blend on high speed until smooth, about 1 minute.

2. Transfer to an airtight container and store in the refrigerator for up to 1 week or freeze in 2-tablespoon servings (use an ice-cube tray) for up to 6 months.

Variation Tip *You can replace the parsley with a green veggie such as spinach or kale. If you're not sensitive to nightshades, consider adding a pinch of red pepper flakes to punch up the flavor even more. You can also use orange zest in place of the lemon zest.*

PER 2 TABLESPOONS Calories: 237; Total Fat: 26g; Saturated Fat: 4g; Cholesterol: 0mg; Carbohydrates: 4g; Fiber: 2g; Protein: 1g

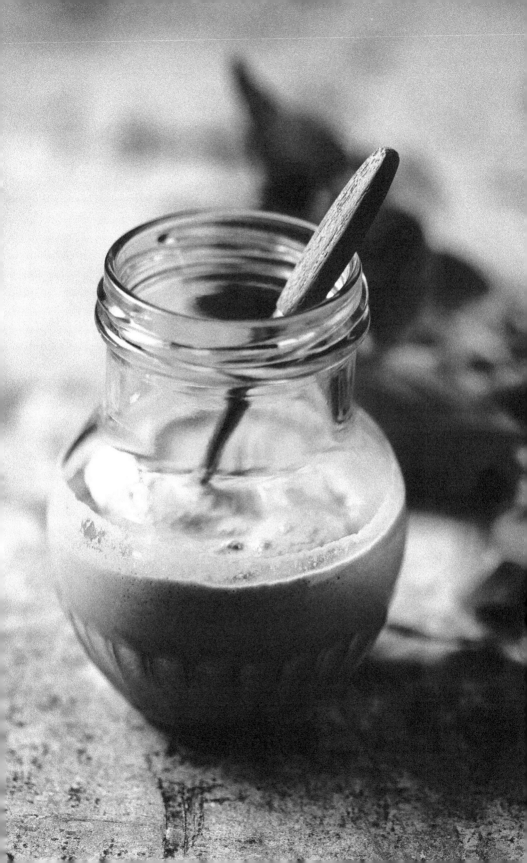

GUACAMOLE

....

YIELD: 1½ CUPS · PREP TIME: 10 MINUTES · COOK TIME: NONE

This is a chunky guacamole that is a great accompaniment for many foods. I like scooping a bit on top of chili, topping a hamburger patty, using it as a veggie dip, or even eating it in the morning with my bacon and eggs. As a much-loved condiment, I've found dozens of ways to use it over the years. When storing, put the plastic wrap directly on the surface of the guacamole to keep air from oxidizing the avocados.

2 avocados, peeled, pitted, and cubed

½ red onion, finely chopped

2 tablespoons apple cider vinegar

2 garlic cloves, minced

Zest of 1 lime

¼ teaspoon ground cumin

3 tablespoons chopped fresh cilantro leaves (optional)

1. In a small bowl, combine all of the ingredients.
2. Using a fork, mash the ingredients together to the desired consistency.

Ingredient Tip *Not everyone likes the taste of cilantro. Some people have a gene that causes this herb to taste "soapy." If you're one of those people, feel free to skip the soap. If you tolerate citrus, replace the apple cider vinegar with the juice of 1 lime.*

PER 2 TABLESPOONS Calories: 72; Total Fat: 7g; Saturated Fat: 1g; Cholesterol: 0mg; Carbohydrates: 4g; Fiber: 2g; Protein: <1g

EASY MAYONNAISE

....

YIELD: 1 CUP · PREP TIME: 10 MINUTES · COOK TIME: NONE

Mayonnaise is really easy to make, and with homemade mayo, you can control the ingredients. Commercial mayonnaise often has sugar, corn syrup, or similar ingredients. Mayo is just an emulsion of egg yolk, vinegar, and oil. I like to make mine using half avocado oil and half extra-virgin olive oil, because mayo made 100 percent with the latter has too strong an olive oil taste. The avocado oil neutralizes it somewhat, while still leaving the character of the olive oil intact.

1 egg yolk

2 teaspoons red wine vinegar

¼ teaspoon Dijon mustard

½ teaspoon sea salt

½ cup extra-virgin olive oil

½ cup avocado oil

1. In a food processor or blender, combine the egg yolk, red wine vinegar, mustard, and salt. Blend on high speed for 10 seconds, or until mixed.

2. In a glass measuring cup, mix the olive oil and avocado oil.

3. With the food processor or blender running, start adding the oil, 1 drop at a time for 10 drops and then in a very thin stream until all of the oil is incorporated.

4. Store in a covered container in the refrigerator for up to 5 days.

Variation Tip Make garlic aioli by adding 2 minced garlic cloves to the blender when you add the egg yolk, and then continuing with the recipe as written. You can also get fancy by adding all sorts of other herbs to the mayonnaise in the first step.

PER 2 TABLESPOONS Calories: 134; Total Fat: 15g; Saturated Fat: 2g; Cholesterol: 26mg; Carbohydrates: <1g; Fiber: <1g; Protein: <1g

PICKLED RED ONIONS

YIELD: 1 CUP · PREP TIME: 5 MINUTES, PLUS 2 HOURS TO MARINATE · COOK TIME: NONE

Pickled red onions are a great condiment for burgers and salads, or in the Gyro Salad (page 208). In fact, my husband refuses to eat gyros unless there are pickled onions and garlic aïoli on the side, and I'm happy to accommodate him. These are so easy to make— as easy as slicing onions, pouring on some vinegar, and sitting back to wait. These will keep in the refrigerator for up to 1 week.

1 cup red wine vinegar

1 teaspoon sea salt

1 drop liquid stevia

½ red onion, thinly sliced

1. In a small bowl, whisk together the vinegar, salt, and stevia until the salt dissolves.

2. Add the onion and submerge it in the vinegar. If needed, add more vinegar to completely cover the onions. Cover and refrigerate for at least 2 hours.

Variation Tip *You can do this kind of quick pickle with cucumbers as well. They won't be the same as store-bought dill pickles, but the vinegar and crisp, fresh cucumber make a wonderful condiment or salad topping.*

PER ½ CUP Calories: 18; Total Fat: 0g; Saturated Fat: 0g; Cholesterol: 0mg; Carbohydrates: 2g; Fiber: <1g; Protein: <1g

CARAMELIZED ONIONS

....

YIELD: 2 CUPS · PREP TIME: 5 MINUTES · COOK TIME: 30 MINUTES

Caramelized onions have a deeply savory flavor (called umami) that can add depth to soups and stews, or ramp up the taste of burgers or other cuts of animal protein. They're great in a frittata or omelet as well. I like to cook large batches of caramelized onions and freeze 1-cup portions in zipper-close bags, ready to be pulled out whenever I think I need a little extra "something" in a dish.

3 tablespoons extra-virgin olive oil

3 yellow onions, sliced

1 teaspoon sea salt

½ teaspoon dried thyme

1. In a Dutch oven over medium-high heat, heat the olive oil until it shimmers.

2. Add the onions, salt, and thyme and cook for 3 minutes, or until the onions begin to soften.

3. Reduce the heat to low. Cook, stirring occasionally, for 30 minutes, or until the onions are a deep mahogany color and have significantly reduced in size and moisture.

4. Store, tightly sealed, in the refrigerator for up to 5 days or in the freezer for up to 1 year.

Ingredient Tip *You can use any type of onion, although Spanish and yellow onions produce the best flavor. Sweet onions, such as Walla Walla or Vidalia, tend to be much sweeter when caramelized, as do red onions. To slice the onions easily, cut off the non-root end (remember to save that end, the peel, and the root end for making stock). Then, halve the onion pole-to-pole (lengthwise), leaving the root end intact. Peel the onion and slice the halves with a very sharp chef's knife.*

PER ¼ CUP Calories: 99; Total Fat: 9g; Saturated Fat: 1g; Cholesterol: 0mg; Carbohydrates: 6g; Fiber: 1g; Protein: <1g

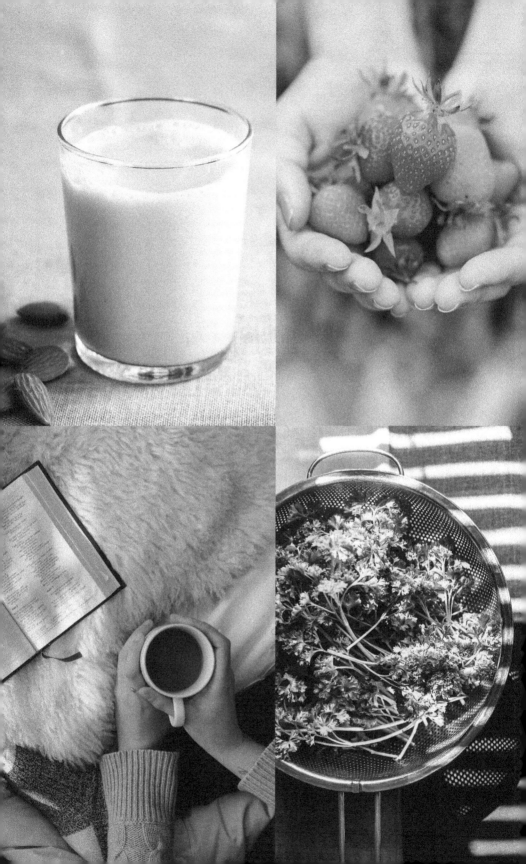

ACKNOWLEDGMENTS

I am really lucky because, professionally, I get to be involved with the things I love the most: writing, cooking, nutrition, and health. Over the years, I have had many helpful mentors in these areas. Thanks to both my mothers, Brenda Riseland and Etta Kirk, for teaching me to cook. Thanks to my husband, Jim, and my boys, Kevin and Tanner, for being my food guinea pigs. I also want to thank Clara Song Lee, my great editor, and Dr. Marybeth Lambe, whose contributions of knowledge were invaluable to the content curation of this book. It has been great to share ideas, and it has enriched my personal Hashimoto's healing journey.

FOODS TO ENJOY, LIMIT, AND AVOID

ANIMAL PROTEINS

Enjoy with Gusto	**May Be Okay for Some**	*Avoid (A) or Limit (L)*
Pastured meats, including:	Fish	Feedlot meats, including:
Beef	Mollusks	Beef (A)
Bison	Shellfish	Bison (A)
Chicken		Chicken (A)
Duck		Eggs (A)
Eggs		Lamb (A)
Game meats		Organ meats (A)
Lamb		Pork (A)
Organ meats		Turkey (A)
Pork		
Turkey		

BEVERAGES

Enjoy with Gusto	**May Be Okay for Some**	*Avoid (A) or Limit (L)*
Herbal tea	Tomato juice	Alcohol (L)
Sparkling water	Vegetable juice	Coffee (caffeinated) (L)
Water		Energy drinks (A)
		Fruit juice (L)
		Soda (regular and diet) (A)
		Sugary beverages (A)
		Tea (caffeinated) (L)

DAIRY/DAIRY REPLACEMENTS

Enjoy with Gusto	May Be Okay for Some	Avoid (A) or Limit (L)
Coconut milk (light and regular)	Almond milk, unsweetened	Butter (A)
Coconut yogurt (plain, unsweetened)	Almond yogurt (plain, unsweetened)	Cheese (A)
Hemp milk, unsweetened		Cheese alternatives (A)
Rice milk, unsweetened		Cream (A)
		Ice cream (A)
		Ice milk (A)
		Milk (A)
		Soymilk (A)
		Soy yogurt (A)
		Yogurt (A)

FATS AND OILS

Enjoy with Gusto	May Be Okay for Some	Avoid (A) or Limit (L)
Animal fats from pastured animals		Animal fats from feedlot animals
Expeller-pressed oils, including:		*Industrial seed oils, including:*
Avocado oil		Butter (L)
Coconut oil		Canola oil (A)
Extra-virgin olive oil		Corn oil (A)
Sesame oil		Light olive oil (A)
		Safflower oil (A)
		Sesame oil (A)
		Soybean oil (A)
		Sunflower oil (A)

FRUITS

Enjoy with Gusto	May Be Okay for Some	Avoid (A) or Limit (L)
Açaí	Citrus fruits	Dried fruits (L)
Apple	Goji berry	Fruit juice, 100% (L)
Avocado	Gooseberry	
Banana	Tomato	
Berries		
Cherries		
Kiwi		
Mango		
Melons		
Nectarine		
Papaya		
Peach		
Pear		
Pineapple		
Plum		
Pluot		

GRAINS

Enjoy with Gusto	May Be Okay for Some	Avoid (A) or Limit (L)
Oats (gluten-free)	Buckwheat	Barley (A)
Rice, brown		Corn (A)
Quinoa		Rice, white (L)
Wild rice		Rye (A)
		Wheat (A)

HERBS, SPICES, AND FLAVORINGS

Enjoy with Gusto	May Be Okay for Some	Avoid (A) or Limit (L)
Apple cider vinegar	Cayenne	Mustard (L)
Allspice	Chili powder	
Anise	Chipotle	
Balsamic vinegar	Paprika	
Black pepper	Sriracha	
Caraway		
Chives		
Cilantro		
Cinnamon		
Cloves		
Coriander		
Cumin		
Fennel seed		
Garlic		
Ginger		
Nutmeg		
Nutritional yeast		
Oregano		
Parsley		
Red wine vinegar		
Rosemary		
Sage		
Sea salt		
Shallot		
Tarragon		
Thyme		
Turmeric		

LEGUMES/PULSES

Enjoy with Gusto	May Be Okay for Some	Avoid (A) or Limit (L)
	Beans (black, kidney, navy, fava, lima, etc.)	Edamame (A)
		Peanuts (A)
	Black-eyed peas	Soy (A)
	Chickpeas	
	Lentils	
	Peas	

NUTS AND SEEDS

Enjoy with Gusto	May Be Okay for Some	Avoid (A) or Limit (L)
Chia	Almonds	Sesame seeds (L)
Coconut	Brazil nuts	
Flaxseed	Cashews	
Hemp seeds	Hazelnuts (filberts)	
Pumpkin seeds	Pecans	
Sunflower seeds	Walnuts	
	Macadamia	

PACKAGED FOODS

Enjoy with Gusto	May Be Okay for Some	Avoid (A) or Limit (L)
Beef stock		Baked goods (A)
Chicken stock		Bread (A)
Frozen fruit (sugar-free)		Canned foods (A)
Frozen vegetables (sugar-free)		Frozen dinners (A)
		Pasta (A)
Turkey stock		Snack foods (A)
Vegetable stock		Tortillas (A)

SUGAR AND SWEETENERS

Enjoy with Gusto	May Be Okay for Some	Avoid (A) or Limit (L)
Stevia	Erythritol	Acesulfame-K (A)
	Mannitol	Aspartame (A)
	Xylitol	Brown sugar (A)
		Corn syrup (A)
		Honey (L)
		Maple syrup, pure (L)
		Molasses (A)
		Saccharine (A)
		Sucralose (A)
		Sugar (A)

VEGETABLES

Enjoy with Gusto	May Be Okay for Some	Avoid (A) or Limit (L)
Arugula	Bell peppers	Bean Sprouts (A)
Asparagus	Chile peppers	Bok choy (L)
Artichoke	Eggplant	Broccoli (L)
Carrots	Potatoes	Broccolini (L)
Celery	Tomatillos	Brussels sprouts (L)
Fennel		Cabbage (L)
Jicama		Cauliflower (L)
Leeks		Chard (L)
Lettuce		Collard greens (L)
Mushrooms		Corn (A)
Onions		Kale (L)
Rutabaga		Mustard greens (L)
Scallions		Radish (L)
Spinach		
Summer squash		
Sweet potato		
Turnips		
Yam		
Winter squash		

THE DIRTY DOZEN
AND THE CLEAN FIFTEEN

A nonprofit environmental watchdog organization called Environmental Working Group (EWG) looks at data supplied by the US Department of Agriculture (USDA) and the Food and Drug Administration (FDA) about pesticide residues. Each year it compiles a list of the best and worst pesticide loads found in commercial crops. You can use these lists to decide which fruits and vegetables to buy organic to minimize your exposure to pesticides and which produce is considered safe enough to buy conventionally. This does not mean they are pesticide-free, though, so wash these fruits and vegetables thoroughly.

These lists change every year, so make sure you look up the most recent one before you fill your shopping cart. You'll find the most recent lists as well as a guide to pesticides in produce at EWG.org/FoodNews.

2015 Dirty Dozen

Apples	Potatoes	*In addition to the Dirty Dozen, the EWG added two types of produce contaminated with highly toxic organo-phosphate insecticides:*
Celery	Snap peas (imported)	
Cherry tomatoes	Spinach	
Cucumbers	Strawberries	
Grapes	Sweet bell peppers	
Nectarines (imported)		Kale/Collard greens
Peaches		Hot peppers

2015 Clean Fifteen

Asparagus	Eggplants	Papayas
Avocados	Grapefruits	Pineapples
Cabbage	Kiwis	Sweet corn
Cantaloupes (domestic)	Mangos	Sweet peas (frozen)
Cauliflower	Onions	Sweet potatoes

CONVERSION TABLES

Volume Equivalents (Liquid)

US STANDARD	US STANDARD (OUNCES)	METRIC (APPROXIMATE)
2 tablespoons	1 fl. oz.	30 mL
¼ cup	2 fl. oz.	60 mL
½ cup	4 fl. oz.	120 mL
1 cup	8 fl. oz.	240 mL
1½ cups	12 fl. oz.	355 mL
2 cups or 1 pint	16 fl. oz.	475 mL
4 cups or 1 quart	32 fl. oz.	1 L
1 gallon	128 fl. oz.	4 L

Oven Temperatures

FAHRENHEIT (F)	CELSIUS (C) (APPROXIMATE)
250°	120°
300°	150°
325°	165°
350°	180°
375°	190°
400°	200°
425°	220°
450°	230°

Volume Equivalents (Dry)

US STANDARD	METRIC (APPROXIMATE)
⅛ teaspoon	0.5 mL
¼ teaspoon	1 mL
½ teaspoon	2 mL
¾ teaspoon	4 mL
1 teaspoon	5 mL
1 tablespoon	15 mL
¼ cup	59 mL
⅓ cup	79 mL
½ cup	118 mL
⅔ cup	156 mL
¾ cup	177 mL
1 cup	235 mL
2 cups or 1 pint	475 mL
3 cups	700 mL
4 cups or 1 quart	1 L

Weight Equivalents

US STANDARD	METRIC (APPROXIMATE)
½ ounce	15 g
1 ounce	30 g
2 ounces	60 g
4 ounces	115 g
8 ounces	225 g
12 ounces	340 g
16 ounces or 1 pound	455 g

REFERENCES

American Autoimmune Related Diseases Association. "Autoimmune Statistics." Accessed December 29, 2015. www.aarda.org/autoimmune-information/autoimmune-statistics/.

American Psychological Association. "How Stress Affects Your Health." Accessed December 29, 2015. www.apa.org/helpcenter/stress.aspx.

American Thyroid Association. "Iodine Deficiency." Accessed December 29, 2015. www.thyroid.org/iodine-deficiency.

American Thyroid Association. "Thyroid Hormone Therapy." *Clinical Thyroidology for Patients* 1, no. 1 (2015): 21. www.thyroid.org/patient-thyroid-information/ct-for-patients/vol-1-issue-1/vol-1-issue-1-p-21/.

Arthur, John R., and Geoffrey J. Beckett. "Thyroid Function." *British Medical Bulletin* 55, no. 3 (1999): 658–68. bmb.oxfordjournals.org/content/55/3/658.full.pdf.

Awad, A.G. "The Thyroid and the Mind and Emotions/Thyroid Dysfunction and Mental Disorders." Thyroid Foundation of Canada. Accessed December 26, 2015. www.thyroid.ca/e10f.php

Betsy, Ambooken, M.P. Binitha, and S. Sarita. "Zinc Deficiency Associated with Hypothyroidism: An Overlooked Cause of Severe Alopecia." *International Journal of Trichology* 5, no. 1 (January–March 2013): 40–42. doi:10.4103/0974-7753.114714.

CDC Features. "Insufficient Sleep Is a Public Health Problem." Centers for Disease Control and Prevention. Last modified September 3, 2015. www.cdc.gov/features/dssleep/.

Chen, Aimin, Stephani S. Kim, Ethan Chung, and Kim N. Deitch. "Thyroid Hormones in Relation to Lead, Mercury, and Cadmium Exposure in the National Health and Nutrition Examination Survey, 2007–2008." *Environmental Health Perspectives* 121, no. 2 (February 2013). doi:10.1289/ehp.1205239.

Chistiakov, Dimitry A. "Immunogenetics of Hashimoto's Thyroiditis." *Journal of Autoimmune Diseases* 2, No. 1. (March 2005). doi:10.1186/1740-2557-2-1.

Daley, Cynthia A., Amber Abbott, Patrick S. Doyle, Glenn A. Nader, and Stephanie Larson. "A Review of Fatty Acid Profiles and Antioxidant Content in Grass-Fed and Grain-Fed Beef." *Nutrition Journal* 9, no. 10 (March 2010). doi:10.1186/1475-2891-9-10.

Delves, Peter J. "Autoimmune Disorders." *Merck Manual Consumer Version*. Accessed December 29, 2015. www.merckmanuals.com /home/immune-disorders/allergic-reactions-and-other-hypersensitivity-disorders/autoimmune-disorders.

Delves, Peter J. "Overview of the Immune System." *Merck Manual Consumer Version*. Accessed December 29, 2015. www.merckmanuals.com/home/immune-disorders/biology -of-the-immune-system/overview-of-the-immune-system.

Drutel, Anne, Françoise Archambeaud, and Philippe Caron. "Selenium and the Thyroid Gland: More Good News for Clinicians." *Clinical Endocrinology* 78, no. 2 (February 2013): 155–64. doi:10.1111/cen.12066.

Encyclopedia Britannica Online. "Inflammation/Pathology." Accessed December 29, 2015. www.britannica.com/science/inflammation.

"Hashimoto's Disease Fact Sheet (ePublication)." Office on Women's Health, US Department of Health and Human Services. Accessed December 26, 2015. www.womenshealth.gov/publications /our-publications/fact-sheet/hashimoto-disease.pdf

Health Guide. "Chronic Thyroiditis (Hashimoto's Disease)." *New York Times*. Accessed December 29, 2015. www.nytimes.com/health /guides/disease/chronic-thyroiditis-hashimotos-disease /possible-complications.html.

Healthy Sleep. "Sleep and Disease Risk." Division of Sleep Medicine at Harvard Medical School. Last modified December 18, 2007. healthysleep.med.harvard.edu/healthy/matters/consequences /sleep-and-disease-risk.

Holtorf Medical Group. "Is It Mental Illness, or Hashimoto's Disease?" Accessed December 29, 2015. www.holtorfmed.com /mental-illness-hashimotos-disease/.

Jabbar, A., A. Yawar, S. Waseem, N. Islam, N. Ul-Haque, L. Zuberi, A. Khan, and J. Akhter. "Vitamin B12 Deficiency Common in Primary Hypothyroidism." *Journal of Pakistan Medical Association* 58, no. 5 (May 2008): 258–61. www.ncbi.nlm.nih.gov/pubmed/18655403.

Jacob, Agalee. "Gut Health and Autoimmune Disease: Research Suggests Digestive Abnormalities May Be the Underlying Cause." *Today's Dietician* 15, no. 2 (February 2013): 32. www.todaysdietitian.com/newarchives/021313p38.shtml.

Jain, Ram B. "Thyroid Function and Serum Copper, Selenium, and Zinc in General U.S. Population." *Biological Trace Element Research* 159, nos. 1–3 (2014): 87–98. doi:10.1007 /s12011-014-9992-9.

Johnson, Larry E. "Mineral Deficiency and Toxicity: Selenium." *Merck Manual Professional Version.* Accessed December 29, 2015. www.merckmanuals.com/professional/nutritional-disorders /mineral-deficiency-and-toxicity/selenium.

Jones, Jeffrey M. "In U.S., 40% Get Less Than Recommended Amount of Sleep." December 19, 2013. Gallup. www.gallup.com /poll/166553/less-recommended-amount-sleep.aspx.

Katie, Byron. "Do The Work." The Work (blog). Accessed December 29, 2015. thework.com/en/do-work.

Katie, Byron, and Michael Katz. *I Need Your Love: Is That True? How to Stop Seeking Love, Approval, and Appreciation and Start Finding Them Instead.* New York: Harmony, 2005.

Katie, Byron, and Stephen Mitchell. *Loving What Is: Four Questions That Can Change Your Life.* New York: Harmony, 2002.

Kirby, David. "The Nutritional Superiority of Pasture Raised Animals." *Huffington Post.* May 29, 2010. www.huffingtonpost. com/david-kirby/the-nutritional-superiori_b_517707.html.

Kresser, Chris. "Basics of Immune Balancing for Hashimoto's." *Chris Kresser.* August 30, 2010. chriskresser.com/basics-of-immune-balancing-for-hashimotos/.

Kresser, Chris. "Iodine for Hypothyroidism: Crucial Nutrient or Harmful Toxin?" *Chris Kresser.* July 5, 2010. chriskresser.com/iodine-for-hypothyroidism-like-gasoline-on-a-fire/.

Kresser, Chris. "Three Reasons Why Your Thyroid Medication Isn't Working." *Chris Kresser.* July 1, 2010. chriskresser.com/three-reasons-why-your-thyroid-medication-isnt-working/.

Lind, P., W. Langsteger, M. Molnar, H.J. Gallowitsch, P. Mikosch, and I. Gomez. "Epidemiology of Thyroid Diseases in Iodine Sufficiency." *Thyroid* 8, no. 12 (1998): 1179–83. www.ncbi.nlm.nih.gov/pubmed/9920375.

Mackawy, Amal Mohammed Husein, Bushra Mohammed Al-ayed, and Bashayer Mater Al-rashidi. "Vitamin D Deficiency and its Association with Thyroid Disease." *International Journal of Health Sciences* 7, no. 3 (November 2013): 267–75. www.ncbi.nlm.nih.gov/pmc/articles/PMC3921055/.

Mann, Denise. "Alcohol and a Good Night's Sleep Don't Mix." WebMD. January 3, 2013. www.webmd.com/sleep-disorders/news/20130118/alcohol-sleep.

Mayo Clinic. "Hashimoto's Disease: Complications." Accessed December 29, 2015. www.mayoclinic.org/diseases-conditions/hashimotos-disease/basics/complications/con-20030293.

McCullough, Kenneth C., and Artur Summerfield. "Basic Concepts of Immune Response and Defense Development." *ILAR Journal* 46, no. 3 (2005): 230–40. doi:10.1093/ilar.46.3.230.

MedlinePlus. "Autoimmune Disorders." U.S. National Library of Medicine. Last modified July 16, 2013. www.nlm.nih.gov/medlineplus/ency/article/000816.htm.

National Institute of Alcohol Abuse and Alcoholism. "Beyond Hangovers." National Institutes of Health. September 2010. pubs.niaaa.nih.gov/publications/Hangovers/beyondHangovers.htm.

National Institute of Diabetes and Digestive and Kidney Disease. "Hashimoto's Disease." National Institutes of Health. May 2014. www.niddk.nih.gov/health-information/health-topics /endocrine/hashimotos-disease/Pages/fact-sheet.aspx.

Neff, Kristin. *Self-Compassion: Stop Beating Yourself Up and Leave Insecurity Behind.* New York: William Morrow, 2011.

Nekrasova, T.A., L.G. Strongin, and O.V. Ledentsova. "Hematological Disturbances in Subclinical Hypothyroidism and Their Dynamics during Substitution Therapy." *Klinicheskaia Meditsina* 91 no. 9 (2013): 29–33. www.ncbi.nlm.nih.gov/pubmed/24437152.

Nordqvist, Christian. "What Is Hashimoto's Thyroiditis or Hashimoto's Disease?" Medical News Today. Last modified September 12, 2014. www.medicalnewstoday.com/articles/266780.php.

Office of Dietary Supplements. "Vitamin D." National Institutes of Health. Accessed December 29, 2015. ods.od.nih.gov/factsheets /VitaminD-HealthProfessional/.

PubMed Health. "How Does the Thyroid Work?" U.S. National Library of Medicine. Last modified January 7, 2015. www.ncbi.nlm.nih.gov /pubmedhealth/PMH0072572/.

Rattue, Grace. "Autoimmune Disease Rates Increasing." Medical News Today. June 22, 2012. www.medicalnewstoday.com /articles/246960.php.

Refaat, Bassem. "Prevalence and Characteristics of Anemia Associated with Thyroid Disorders in Non-pregnant Saudi Women during the Childbearing Age: A Cross-sectional Study." *Biomedical Journal* 38, no. 4 (July–August 2015): 307–16. doi:10.4103/2319-4170.151032.

Sathyapalan, Thozhukat, Alireza M. Manuchehri, Natalie J. Thatcher, Alan S. Rigby, Tom Chapman, Eric S. Kilpatrick, and Stephen L. Atkin. "The Effect of Soy Phytoestrogen Supplementation on Thyroid Status and Cardiovascular Risk Markers in Patients with Subclinical Hypothyroidism: A Randomized, Double-Blind, Crossover Study." *Journal of Clinical Endocrinology & Metabolism* 96, no. 5 (May 2011): 1442–49. doi:10.1210/jc.2010-2255.

Sicherer, Scott H., Anne Muñoz-Furlong, and Hugh A. Sampson. "Prevalence of Seafood Allergy in the United States Determined by a Random Telephone Survey." *Journal of Allergy and Clinical Immunology* 114, no. 1 (July 2004):159–65. www.ncbi.nlm.nih.gov /pubmed/15241360.

Somers, Emily C., Martha A. Ganser, Jeffrey S. Warren, Niladri Basu, Lu Wang, Suzanna M. Zick, and Sung Kyun Park. "Mercury Exposure and Antinuclear Antibodies among Females of Reproductive Age in the United States: NHANES." *Environmental Health Perspectives* 123, no. 8 (August 2015). doi:10.1289/ehp.1408751.

Sutherland, Stephani. "Bright Screens Could Delay Bedtime." *Scientific American.* January 1, 2013. www.scientificamerican.com /article/bright-screens-could-delay-bedtime/.

Thorpy, Michael. "Sleep Hygiene." *National Sleep Foundation.* Accessed December 29, 2015. sleepfoundation.org/ask-the-expert /sleep-hygiene.

U.S. Food and Drug Administration. "What You Need to Know About Mercury in Fish and Shellfish (Brochure)." Accessed December 29, 2015. www.fda.gov/food/resourcesforyou /consumers/ucm110591.htm.

Vanderpump, Mark P.J. "The Epidemiology of Thyroid Disease." *British Medical Bulletin* 99, no. 1 (June 2011). doi10.1093/bmb/ldr030.

Van Donkersgoed, Joyce, Valerie Bohaychuk, Thomas Besser, Xin-Ming Song, Bruce Wagner, Dale Hancock, David Renter, and David Dargatz. "Occurrence of Foodborne Bacteria in Alberta Feedlots." *Canadian Veterinary Journal* 50, no. 2 (February 2009): 166–72. www.ncbi.nlm.nih.gov/pmc/articles/PMC2629420/.

WebMD. "What Is Inflammation?" Accessed December 29, 2015. www.webmd.com/arthritis/about-inflammation.

Womenshealth.gov. "Hashimoto's Disease Fact Sheet." Office on Women's Health, U.S. Department of Health & Human Services. Accessed December 29, 2015. womenshealth.gov/publications /our-publications/fact-sheet/hashimoto-disease.html.

Xue, Haibo, Weiwei Wang, Yuanbin Li, Zhongyan Shan, Yushu Li, Xiaochun Teng, Yun Gao, C. Fan, and W. Teng. "Selenium Upregulates CD4 CD25 Regulatory T Cells in Iodine-induced Autoimmune Thyroiditis Model of NOD.H-2h4 Mice." *Endocrine Journal* 57, no. 7 (April 2010): 595–601. www.ncbi.nlm.nih.gov /pubmed/20453397?dopt=AbstractPlus.

Yoon, Soo-Jee, So-Rae Choi, Dol-Mi Kim, Jun-Uh Kim, Kyung-Wook Kim, Chul-Woo Ahn, et al. "The Effect of Iodine Restriction on Thyroid Function in Patients with Hypothyroidism Due to Hashimoto's Thyroiditis." *Yonsei Medical Journal* 44, no. 2 (April 2003): 227–35. www.ncbi.nlm.nih.gov/pubmed/12728462.

Zimmermann, Michael B., and Josef Köhrle. "The Impact of Iron and Selenium Deficiencies on Iodine and Thyroid Metabolism: Biochemistry and Relevance to Public Health." *Thyroid* 12, no. 10 (October 2002): 867–78. www.ncbi.nlm.nih.gov /pubmed/12487769.

RESOURCES

Books and Publications

Frazier, Karen. *Hashimoto's Cookbook and Action Plan: 31 Days to Eliminate Toxins and Restore Thyroid Health Through Diet.* Berkeley, CA: Rockridge Press, 2015.

Katie, Byron. *I Need Your Love: Is That True? How to Stop Seeking Love, Approval, and Appreciation, and Start Finding Them Instead.* New York: Harmony Books, 2005.

Katie, Byron. *Loving What Is: Four Questions That Can Change Your Life.* New York: Harmony Books, 2002.

Neff, Kristin. *Self-Compassion: The Proven Power of Being Kind to Yourself.* New York: William Morrow, 2014

Rosenberg, Marshall B. *Nonviolent Communication: A Language of Life.* Encinitas, CA: PuddleDancer Press, 2003

Websites

Celiac.com: celiac.com

EndocrineWeb: endocrineweb.com

Self-Compassion/Dr. Kristin Neff: self-compassion.org

Stop the Thyroid Madness: stopthethyroidmadness.com

Women's Health: womenshealth.gov

The Work of Byron Katie: thework.com

Experts and Organizations

American Autoimmune-Related Diseases Association, Inc.: aarda.org

Functional Medicine Specialist, Chris Kresser: chriskresser.com

National Sleep Foundation: sleepfoundation.org

Thyroid Foundation of Canada: thyroid.ca

RECIPE INDEX

INDEX

foods. *See also* canned foods;
    packaged foods
  to enjoy, 73
  reintroducing, 74–75
freezer, using, 125
fried eggs, 186–187. *See also* eggs
fries, as snack, 154
frittata, mushroom, 141
fruits. *See also* citrus fruits
  avoiding, 242
  enjoying, 69–70, 242
  nutrient-dense, 54
  salad, 160
FT3 (Free T3) and FT4 (Free T4)
    tests, 36

G

garlic
  aioli with scallops, 218–219
  in snack, 152
  and spinach zucchini ribbons,
    174–175
gelatin, in snack, 149
gender, 26
generic medications, 42
genetic component, 24
ginger
  and cilantro vinaigrette, 231
  with pork meatballs, 202–203
  in salad, 157, 162
  in smoothie, 147
gluten grains, avoiding or limiting,
    65–66
goitrogens, minimizing intake of, 54
grains
  avoiding and reintroducing, 71
  avoiding or limiting, 65–66
  enjoying and avoiding, 242
  stocking pantry with, 130
Graves' disease, 22
green beans with scallops, 218–219
green smoothie, 146
ground beef. *See also* beef stew
  and asparagus stir-fry, 207
  in soup, 170–171

H

halibut with dill and zucchini, 212
hash browns, 184–185

Hashimoto, Hakaru, 14
Hashimoto's thyroiditis
  chronic dysfunction, 31–37
  coexisting conditions, 23
  diagnosis, 33
  as "invisible illness," 30
  lack of treatment, 32–33
  statistics, 14
  triggers, 24–28
healthcare providers, 43–45
herbs
  avoiding and reintroducing, 71–72
  enjoying and avoiding, 243
  stocking pantry with, 129
hormones, 19, 22. *See also* NDT
    (natural desiccated thyroid)
humanity, relating to, 86
hummus, as snack, 155

I

immersion blender, 126
immune response, 15
immune system
  autoimmune disease, 16–17
  clean feeding, 53–54
  inflammation, 16–17
  white blood cells, 16
inflammation, 16–17
inner critic, dealing with, 85, 87–88
interventions, trying, 47
iodine, as trigger, 25–26
iron intake, 55–56

J

Jarisch-Herxheimer reaction, 94
jicama, in dip, 153
julienne cutter, 126–127

K

knives, keeping sharp, 127
Kresser, Chris, 56

L

labs, advocating for, 34–35
lamb
  in Gyro Salad, 208
  herb-rubbed, 209
  in soup, 163
leaky gut syndrome, 26–27
leftovers, planning for, 125

ABOUT THE AUTHOR

KAREN FRAZIER is a freelance writer and cookbook author who specializes in writing recipes and meal plans for restrictive diets. She was a personal trainer before Hashimoto's thyroiditis changed her life and led her to adopt a modified diet. Currently she practices Usui Reiki and numerous alternative healing techniques, including aromatherapy and crystal healing. She is the author of *The Hashimoto's Cookbook and Action Plan* and has blogged about her experiences with Hashimoto's on www.karenfrazierblogs.com. She lives with her husband near Seattle.

CPSIA information can be obtained
at www.ICGtesting.com
Printed in the USA
JSHW042252070822
28904JS00001B/1